FOUNDATIO

YOGA FLOW

Collette Ouseley-Moynan
Weston Carls

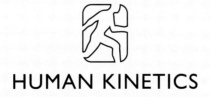

HUMAN KINETICS

Library of Congress Cataloging-in-Publication Data

Names: Ouseley-Moynan, Collette, 1983- author. | Carls, Weston, 1985-
author.
Title: Foundational yoga flow / Collette Ouseley-Moynan, Weston Carls.
Description: Champaign, IL : Human Kinetics, [2025] | Includes
bibliographical references.
Identifiers: LCCN 2024008748 (print) | LCCN 2024008749 (ebook) | ISBN
9781718228092 (print) | ISBN 9781718228108 (epub) | ISBN 9781718228115
(pdf)
Subjects: LCSH: Hatha yoga--Popular works. | BISAC: HEALTH & FITNESS / Yoga
| SPORTS & RECREATION / Training
Classification: LCC RA781.7 .O97 2025 (print) | LCC RA781.7 (ebook) | DDC
613.7/046--dc23/eng/20240405
LC record available at https://lccn.loc.gov/2024008748
LC ebook record available at https://lccn.loc.gov/2024008749

ISBN: 978-1-7182-2809-2 (print)

The web addresses cited in this text were current as of January 2024, unless otherwise noted.

Senior Acquisitions Editor: Michelle Earle; **Developmental Editor:** Amy Stahl; **Managing Editor:** Hannah Werner; **Copyeditor:** Peggy Currid; **Senior Graphic Designer:** Sean Roosevelt; **Cover Designers:** Keri Evans and Weston Carls; **Cover Design Specialist:** Susan Rothermel Allen; **Photographs (cover and interior):** © Human Kinetics/Weston Carls; **Photo Production Specialist:** Amy M. Rose; **Photo Production Manager:** Jason Allen; **Printer:** Versa Press

We thank Monahans Sandhills State Park in Monahans, Texas, and Shafter, Texas, for graciously allowing us to photograph our yoga poses at their locations for this book and to Jim and Jim for allowing us to use their garden and for their boundless Marfa, Texas, knowledge.

Human Kinetics books are available at special discounts for bulk purchase. Special editions or book excerpts can also be created to specification. For details, contact the Special Sales Manager at Human Kinetics.

Printed in the United States of America   10   9   8   7   6   5   4   3   2   1

The paper in this book is certified under a sustainable forestry program.

Human Kinetics
1607 N. Market Street
Champaign, IL 61820
USA

United States and International
Website: **US.HumanKinetics.com**
Email: info@hkusa.com
Phone: 1-800-747-4457

Canada
Website: **Canada.HumanKinetics.com**
Email: info@hkcanada.com

E9502

For my Aunt Johanna: a warrior in action, a poet at heart, and a gift to the world (especially mine). And for my husband, Chris, the yin to my yang.
    —Collette Ouseley-Moynan

To my dog, Teddy, my bodhisattva.
    —Weston Carls

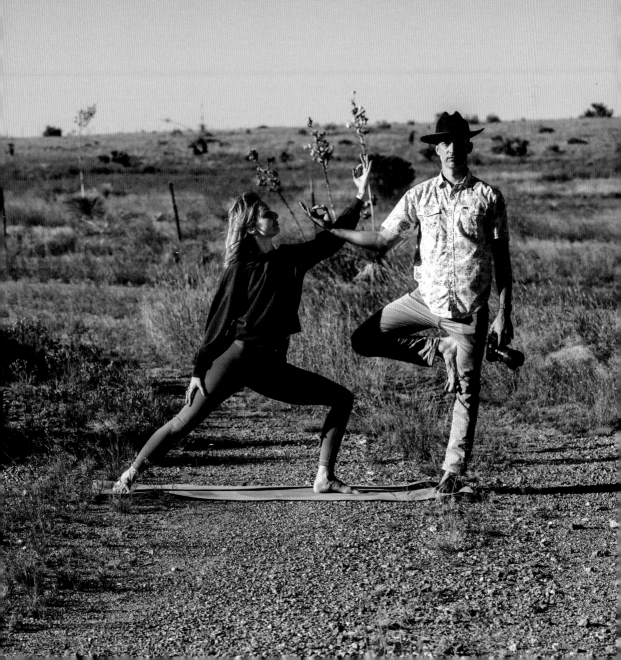

CONTENTS

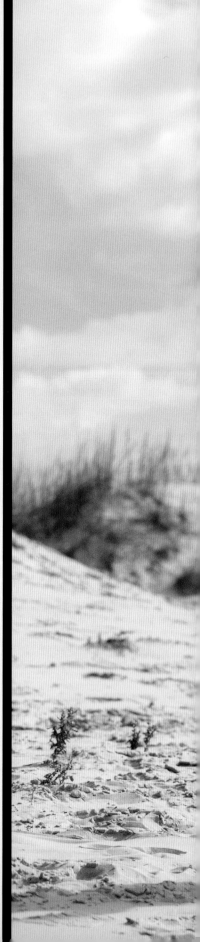

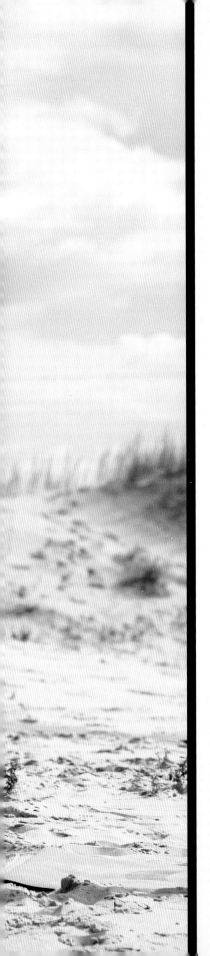

FOREWORD

To say that yoga changed my life would be an understatement. In truth, it would not be an overstatement to say that yoga *saved* my life over a quarter of a century ago. To this day, it remains a sanctuary—a source of connection, strength, and immense joy.

My first yoga practice was with a VHS videotape called *Yoga for Beginners* by Patricia Walden—it was 1996. I remember that about 20 minutes into the class she had us in a pose and said, "Feel the strength and confidence of Warrior II." I had never been in the shape before and really had no idea what I was doing, but when she said those words, I felt *exactly* that: strong and confident. As I stood in the shape, arms stretched wide from side to side, steady in my legs, attention on my breath and my mind focused, I remembered who I was.

That spark of recognition was undeniable. A door had been opened for me, and I was ready to walk through. I began practicing yoga every day; I sought out a teacher and learned to meditate. As my body and mind became both stronger and more flexible, I found a new sense of direction—rather than fearing change, I learned to embrace it.

Feeling at home in our bodies, being connected to our breath, becoming present to ourselves and what we know in our bones—this is the simple yet profound practice we call *yoga*. We do this practice to undo the things that keep us limited and small.

The passion I felt then for yoga is what I still feel today as I step onto my mat or into the yoga classroom. Every time I practice yoga, something *happens*. This simple act of moving the body through shapes with mindfulness and attention to breath *always* delivers. I know this in my own experience, and I see it in my students.

The practice itself is simple, adaptable, and open to innovation. It is our participation that brings yoga to life. Yoga is beyond simply making shapes. It is about bringing our full presence into our bodies within these shapes, deepening connection to our breath, and letting go of worries, tension, and stress. Yoga is the act of becoming our truest selves by shedding the layers of who we are not. It is a way of coming home.

There is a popular saying in the world of yoga: "When the student is ready, the teacher appears." If you are holding this book, it is because you are ready. And you have found a wonderful teacher here in these pages.

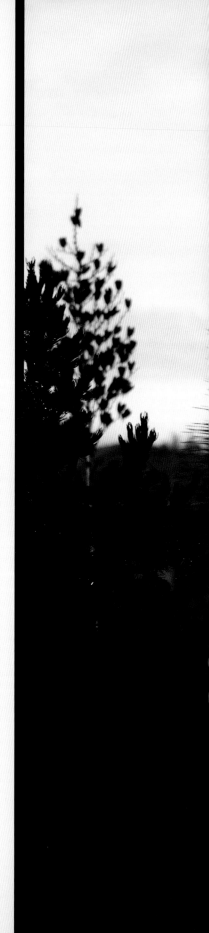

I have known Collette for almost 15 years, and it has been my honor and privilege to be her teacher and mentor. From the beginning, her sincerity and openness as a student were evident, and it has been a joy to teach alongside her in various trainings as she continues to grow in both her practice and teaching.

Collette's sincere love of beauty and art complements her passion for education and her dedication to making yoga accessible to all. From the West Texas landscapes to the real-life yogis you see on these pages, this offering is from the heart. The sequences provide a variety of shapes and options, meeting you where you are each day, as a good yoga practice should. Weston's photography captures more than just poses—he has captured the mood and energy of yogis in practice. Each image is an invitation to step onto your mat and join.

In *Foundational Yoga Flow*, you will find the tools to build a practice that becomes your own place of strength and refuge. This book invites you to explore and embrace your journey. Let each pose be a stepping stone to self-discovery, a beacon guiding you back to your essence. Let the rhythm of your breath be the music that serenades your soul, and let the practice be a dance that brings you home, again and again, to the truth of who you are. Welcome to your practice—welcome home.

Gioconda Parker
Yoga Teacher and Trainer
Spiritual Psychologist and Somatic Experiencing Practitioner
Lover of Life and All Things Yoga (and My Sweet Dog Ash)

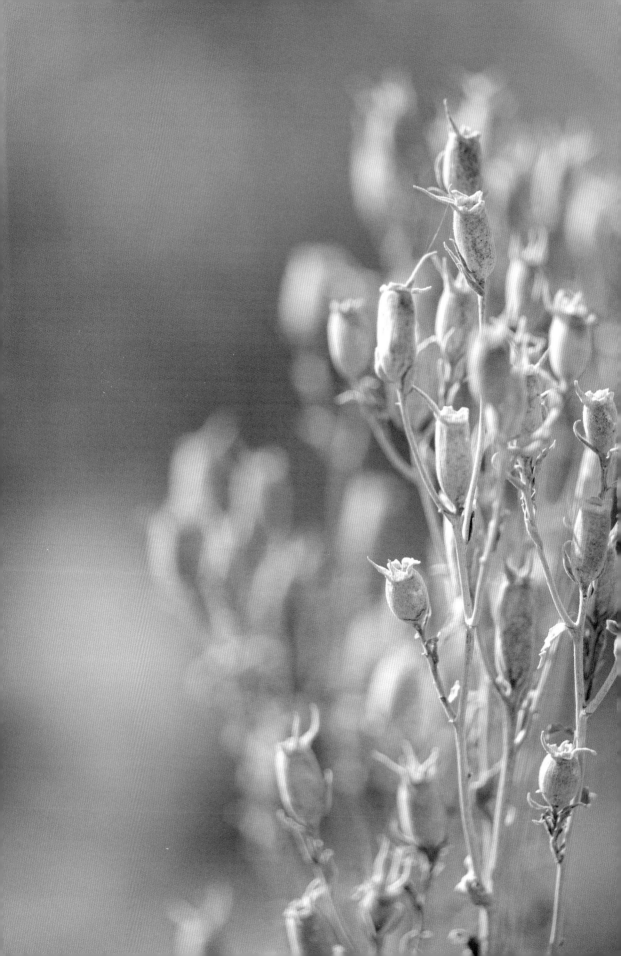

ACKNOWLEDGMENTS

Weston and Collette would like to acknowledge Lauren Brown for her contributions to this book and for helping to ignite this project. They would also like to extend deep gratitude to the crew of models: Abby Sharp, Adam DiMarco, Baldo Garza, and Brooke Wilson.

Weston would like to thank Shelby Autrey for introducing him to yoga. He thanks Leah Cullis for believing in him to photograph her book, *Power Yoga: Strength, Sweat, and Spirit,* and Christine Fenerty for recommending him to photograph David Kyle's book, *Rocket Yoga.* Thanks also to Michelle Earle for giving him creative freedom for this book, *Foundational Yoga Flow.* He would also like to thank Brian Fitzsimmons for his photography mentorship. Thanks to Camp Gladiator for mistaking him as a photographer before he was one, launching his career in fitness photography. Lastly, Weston would like to thank his family for encouraging and supporting him throughout his budding entrepreneurship. Without their help, he wouldn't have endured beyond 2020.

Collette would like to thank the teachers and colleagues who've inspired her teaching through the years—namely, Sam Rice, Mary Dana Abbott, Erinn Leigh, and Justin Ifill—with special acknowledgment for her mentor and friend, Gioconda Parker, for her longtime guidance and cheerleading. Thanks also to Ilana Nankin and the Breathe For Change team for the opportunity to grow with them as a trainer and leader. Finally, she would like to offer deep gratitude to the Castle Hill Fitness community for over a decade of unwavering kindness and support; it is an honor to be a part of the sangha.

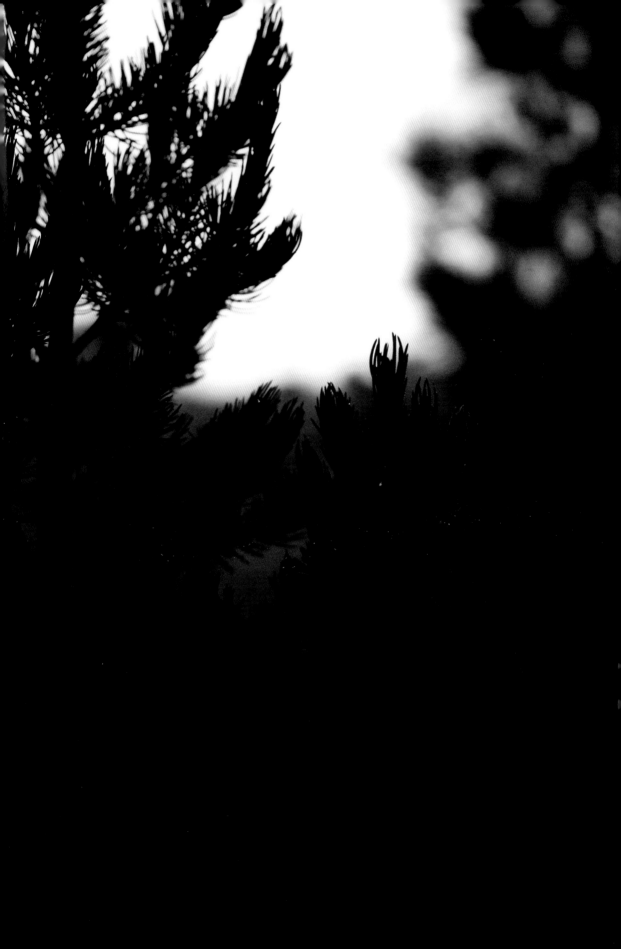

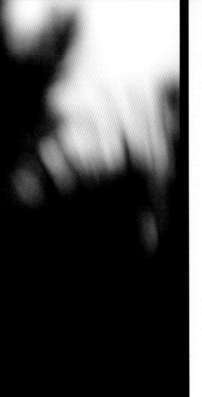

INTRODUCTION

As a child, I loved to move my body—whether in dance class or riding my bike, roller skating, or attempting "gymnastics" on the jungle gym at recess. But I never considered myself athletic. I've never played sports competitively (and yes, I tried out for a few in high school but never made the team). Somewhere along the line, I adopted the story about myself that I was uncoordinated and not strong, so I began to shy away from much physical activity.

When I was in college, a friend convinced me to attend a community yoga class on campus, and I left feeling calmer and more focused. Over the years, I dabbled in yoga and tried various styles and teachers, but it was when I moved to Austin, Texas, in 2009 after finishing my master's in curriculum and instructional leadership that yoga became a lifeline for me. I was having a difficult time adjusting to being in a new city on my own and had relocated during a hiring freeze in the public school system (at the time, I was an elementary school teacher) and was unable to find work.

During this time of transition and uncertainty, my yoga mat became a place of solace and comfort. I could temporarily turn off my anxiety and let go of the weight of an unknown future. I could instead allow my mind to settle on the present moment of being on my mat and in my body. Through the practice, I reconnected with myself on many different levels and started rewriting the story I had mentally composed about living in my body. Instead of thinking I was uncoordinated, I began to trust my balance and ability to move with grace. Instead of believing I was weak, I learned to trust my physical strength, which led me to trust my mental and spiritual strength, too. I began untangling the attachment I had to perfectionism and became willing to take more risks on my mat and to try new things without expectation of the outcome. The work I was doing on the mat had a profound effect on how I was showing up in my life off the mat; this was powerful stuff!

I wanted to share with others the tools I had acquired through yoga—and so began my journey into teaching. Since becoming certified in 2010, I have been teaching yoga and meditation classes and leading 200-hour yoga teacher training courses all over the United States. I've had the pleasure of working with a wide variety of practitioners, from toddlers to octogenarians. Yoga is a practice I've shared with athletes recovering from injury and celebrities recovering from addiction. It has been my sincere pleasure to share in the journey of yoga with my students throughout the years, and I am so grateful to have found this path as both a teacher and a student.

Yoga is a rich practice with a deep history, and it goes far beyond the asana (yoga poses). While this book focuses primarily on the physical aspects of yoga, it is my intention to offer an introduction to the history and philosophy of yoga as a means to inspire you to seek out further teachings and listen to your own innate wisdom as you develop or deepen your practice.

Our Mission

Whether you are beginning your yoga practice or returning to your foundation, the purpose of this book is to be accessible yet aspirational—but ultimately practical. The essence of yoga is connecting to both your own true nature and to the nature of the surrounding universe.

In this book, you'll find images of West Texas that will transport you into the natural world. From the rolling dunes of Monahans Sandhills State Park to the desolate ghost town of Shafter to the grandeur of the Chinati Mountain Range, we invite you to reflect on and enjoy places of great beauty and inspiration. We felt these open, vast, and awe-inspiring places were the perfect backdrop to showcase the wonders of yoga asana, given that many yoga poses are named for and representative of the natural world.

With our team of yogis, Weston and I ventured out to West Texas on a bright and sunny November weekend simply seeking spaces that we were drawn to and that we felt energetically connected with the poses. Just as each place we visited held its own special energy and physical beauty, each asana in each different body radiates its own energy and beauty. Through our photographs, we aim to capture the awe of the natural world (including the human body!) at the time of day in which it was photographed. We also acknowledge and honor the body's corresponding need for both activation and rest throughout the day. You will notice that the poses featured within begin with those that ground and wake up the body and were captured during sunrise. We then move into more vigorous, energizing, and heat-building poses that were shot at the peak of the day. Finally, we close with restorative and passive postures captured beneath a star-filled sky.

We invite you to use this book as a resource and a guide to learn more about the practice of yoga and some of its history and philosophy. Through the photographs and descriptions of the postures, we hope to demystify the practice of yoga asana, and we encourage you to begin or to deepen your physical practice. Most important, we hope to remind you that your yoga practice will be your own—unique to your body—and will likely ebb and flow in how it looks, depending on the season of the year and the season of your life. Yoga asana might feel challenging or too strenuous some days, and we encourage you to remember the restorative poses offered in this book as a complete practice unto themselves. Your body is inherently wise: Listen to the cues and information that arise intuitively as you practice and make adjustments that feel right to you.

This book is a way to enjoy the beauty of asana captured in a moment in time in breathtaking places, and we hope it finds a space on your coffee table and continues to inspire you for years to come!

So, What Is Yoga?

Atha yoga anushasanam: "Now, we begin the study of yoga." This is the first passage in the *Yoga Sutras of Patanjali*, a text believed to have been first codified between the second and fourth centuries BC. It is a reminder that yoga is a practice done in the present moment. Wherever you are, with or without a yoga mat, if you are present in your awareness, your breath, your body, your surroundings—you indeed are practicing yoga.

Yoga is a Sanskrit word that comes from the root word *yuj*, which can be translated to mean "to yoke" or "to unite." Yoga is a practice of uniting the mind with the body. Yoga can bring our self (our egoic mind and awareness) back in connection with our Self (our spirit or higher consciousness). Yoga reminds us of our connection to one another, to all other beings, to this planet, and to the bigger universe. And while we can only ever practice yoga in the now, yoga reminds us of our connection to our past—our roots and our lineage—and invites us to be more aware of and intentional about how we choose to move into the future.

Yoga originated in what is known today as India and was first mentioned in the sacred text the *Rig Veda* around 5,000 years ago (although some historians believe yoga could have originated closer to 10,000 years ago). In the *Bhagavad Gita* (dating back to the sixth through third centuries BC), we are introduced to the four paths, or margas, of yoga that are said to lead to liberation, also referred to as *moksha*:

- Karma yoga (from the root word *kri*, meaning "action"): the path of service and doing good without expectation or attachment to the result of these actions
- Jnana yoga (meaning "wisdom"): the study of ancient texts and philosophy along with the practice of meditation, self-study, and deep inquiry into the nature of who we are
- Bhakti yoga (from the root word *bhaj*, meaning "to bind"): the practice of love and devotion for and of "binding" with the divine through prayer, worship, offerings, ceremonies, and chanting mantras
- Raja yoga (translating to "royal path"): often referred to as the supreme path to moksha, raja yoga presents an eight-step system (which was organized in the *Yoga Sutras of Patanjali*) referring to both the outcome of yoga (enlightenment) and the method of attaining it

Around the 15th century, a sage by the name of Swami Svatmarma composed one of the most influential surviving texts on hatha yoga, called the *Hatha Yoga Pradipika*. This title essentially breaks down to mean "to shed light on the union of the sun and the moon." To refine this definition even further, the text sheds light on how to unite the energies of the masculine (sun) and the feminine (moon) in each of us as a means to achieve higher consciousness. When we refer to hatha yoga today, we mean to unite body and mind through a physical practice that allows for greater clarity and connection.

The postures set forth in the *Hatha Yoga Pradipika* would later evolve into a larger collection of 122 yoga poses called the *Sritattvanidhi*, the first book entirely devoted to asana. This text depicts, for the first time, many postures that we are now familiar with from the ashtanga vinyasa (a style of modern yoga) series and from *Light on Yoga* by B.K.S. Iyengar, a manual of sorts used in most 200-hour yoga teacher trainings across the globe.

Yoga as we now know it in the West can be attributed to the teachings of Tirumalai Krishnamacharya (November 18, 1888–February 28, 1989), considered to be the father of modern yoga. Krishnamacharya cited the *Sritattvanidhi* as a source in his early writings on yoga and drew on this tradition as inspiration while blending it with a number of other sources to systematize the style of hatha vinyasa yoga that most of us are familiar with in the West today. It is said that in 1915, Krishnamacharya ventured to Mount Kailash (considered the eternal abode of the deity Shiva), where he studied asana and pranayama under the tutelage of Sri Ramamohan. In *Health, Healing, and Beyond*, T.K.V. Desikachar (2011; p. 43), son and student of Krishnamacharya, says

> My father once told me that his guru knew about seven thousand asanas. Of these, my father mastered about three thousand. After more than thirty years of study with Krishnamacharya, I know approximately five hundred or so.

This speaks to the breadth of yoga asana and how limited our knowledge of the practice is in modern Western society! When Krishnamacharya left Mount Kailash and the ashram of Sri Ramamohan, he was instructed to bring yoga to the people so that it would be of service to everyday householders and not be reserved only for renunciates living away from society.

Throughout the 1920s, Krishnamacharya traveled throughout India offering lectures and demonstrations of yoga asana. In 1926, upon hearing of Krishnamacharya's skill, the maharaja (prince) of Mysore, India, invited Krishnamacharya to teach yoga to his family at the royal palace. Krishnamacharya further cultivated a style of yoga asana, blending not only the traditional teachings he had received from Sri Ramamohan but also incorporating British gymnastics, martial arts, and military calisthenics. It is important to address that the emphasis on postures and the focus on yoga as a primarily physical practice was born at a time when India was under British colonial rule. When British rule effectively began in 1773, Westerners associated yogis with poverty, witchcraft and black magic, and sexual perversity (based in tantric philosophy), and yogis were relegated to the position of social outcasts. A new merging of traditional hatha yoga with the more Westernized physical fitness—as developed by Krishnamacharya and his students who followed—was considered more palatable when seen through the lens of the West's preference for masculine physicality and feats of strength. While Krishnamacharya never set foot in America, his influence on modern yoga in the West can be found in what comes to mind when we think of "yoga" today, such as sun salutations, vinyasa (linking movement with breath), and even many of the arm balances and inversions that now populate our Instagram feeds.

The Meaning of "Asana"

Asana is a Sanskrit word for "seat"; yoga refers to each posture or shape as a "seat" within the practice. Considering the emphasis that Krishnamacharya and his students—such as B.K.S. Iyengar, K. Pattabhi Jois, and Indra Devi—put on the physical aspect of yoga, it's no surprise that for many of us in the West, when we think of yoga, we think of asana and making shapes with the body. Most practitioners of yoga come upon the practice by hearing about classes focused on movement being offered at their local gym or yoga studio. It's likely that you picked up this book to look at these inspiring and interesting images of various bodies showcasing some of the amazing shapes presented through the practice of yoga asana! While asana is not the be-all and end-all of the yoga practice, we do know that it is through the physical that many people find their way into other aspects of yoga, such as meditation and breath work. With this in mind, we were inspired to create something practical and motivational that would introduce yoga to new practitioners and facilitate a deeper understanding of the anatomy and structure of the postures depicted within for new and seasoned yogis alike.

When it comes to yoga asana, the *Yoga Sutras* set forth by Patanjali offers this directive: "sthira sukham asanam," which translates as "the posture should be a balance of steady and stable effort and comfortable, relaxed engagement." For each of us, at various times of the day and different times in our life, some postures might seem more or less effortful (i.e., challenging) to us than others, and that's perfectly normal! However, within the asana practice, there is an invitation to stay curious about the balance of effort and ease in the shape with each breath that you take. It is through this awareness that we can get closer to balance as we breathe, make adjustments, and invite our mind to settle into the moment.

Yoga Includes Seven Other Limbs

As mentioned previously, the eight-limbed path of yoga Patanjali presented in his *Yoga Sutras* provides a framework, when put into dedicated practice, for finding liberation from physical, mental, and emotional suffering. While presented in a particular order, no one limb takes precedence over another.

Yamas

Yamas are a collection of ethical principles, often referred to as "restraints," that provide a lens through which to see the self and are a means to build the foundation for a healthy and meaningful relationship with the self (and then with others). The yamas are as follows:

- *Ahimsa: nonviolence.* This is a reminder that through kindness and compassion, we can cultivate a loving and caring relationship with our own mind, our emotional experiences, and our bodies that will in turn provide the foundation to live kindly and compassionately in relationship with others.

- *Satya: truthfulness.* We must first be honest with ourselves and live from a place of authenticity to be able to cultivate a meaningful relationship with anyone else.

- *Asteya: nonstealing.* The antidote to feeling envious and lacking, which leads to the act of stealing, is to reflect on the abundance in our lives and to live from a place of gratitude. This includes honoring the body *you* are in and not comparing your practice to anyone else's!

- *Bramacharya: conservation of vital energy.* While Patanjali meant this in reference to abstinence and the conservation of sexual energy, today's yogis can think of this as managing our attention. In this modern world, it's easier than ever to let distractions—like screens, overworking, and poor boundaries with communication devices—take hostage of our time, leaving us feeling disconnected from our bodies and our vitality. Through the practice of bramacharya, we are tasked to be selective with how we spend our time and with whom or what we engage.

- *Aparigraha: nongreed.* This yama asks us to reflect on what we are coveting or chasing and how we become attached to certain outcomes, objects, or statuses. When we can live in flow with life's ups and downs, we will find more ease, acceptance, and peace.

Niyamas

Niyamas, often called disciplines or observances, are a way for the yogi to refine the relationship with the self. The five included by Patanjali are as follows:

- *Saucha: cleanliness.* This applies to your own hygiene and care for your body and being a steward of your space—and the planet!
- *Santosa: contentment and appreciation.* This is not contentment based on getting what you want; it's about finding contentment in being alive.
- *Tapas: discipline.* This literally translates to "to burn," so think of this as pushing through moments of apathy or laziness and staying dedicated to your practice and to your growth and evolution especially when it's challenging.
- *Svadhayaya: self-study.* Looking inwardly with curiosity and learning more about ourselves can give us insight into why we do what we do and how we may be holding ourselves back—like when I believed I was weak. It is also seeking guidance and using tools such as this book to help develop and evolve emotionally, mentally, and spiritually.
- *Isvara pranidhana: devotion and surrender to the supreme.* Patanjali never prescribed a particular higher entity, but recognizing a higher power is a reminder that many things are out of our control. When we trust in forces bigger than our egoic mind, we can release some of our anxieties and attempts at control, with a deep knowing that things will shift and evolve as they are meant to—just like the natural world does season after season.

Pranayama

Pranayama is the practice of working with the breath as a means to regulate the body and the mind. *Prana* translates to "life force," and in yoga, the breath is inextricably connected to vital energy and being alive in the body. Although the breath is part of the autonomic nervous system and is not something we must control, breathing that is intentional, regulated, retained, or extended can have a profound effect on our body, mood, and physical well-being.

Ancient yogis believed that we are born with a finite number of breaths assigned to us by the divine. By learning to control the breath, we can sustain the life force riding the breath as a means to live longer. We do know that the short, shallow, and rapid breath often associated with stress and anxiety is taxing on the body and that deep, diaphragmatic, regulated breathing promotes decreased tension in the body. Therefore, it would make sense that learning to control the breath would indeed promote longevity. The breath, the body, and the mind are in relationship until the final breath we take—by learning to control the breath, even our last one can be deep and easeful, free of anxiety and fear.

Pratyahara

Pratyahara is a practice of turning one's attention inward. Our senses are always providing us with information about the external world. We are often overloaded with external stimuli, which can leave us alternately craving more of the things our senses enjoy or trying to flee the things displeasing to our senses; these external stimuli can have more control over our minds and actions than we may realize. Pratyahara, often called "sense withdrawal," is a practice of sitting with the information coming via the senses without attachment or reaction. As we observe our inner relationship to external stimuli, we become aware of our mind's immediate reaction. We can evaluate, and then we can be more intentional in how we respond to any given situation.

Dharana

Dharana is the practice of concentration. This is the initial step toward meditation, when you begin to settle into a point of focus—such as the breath, the body, a word, or an image. By continuing to return to a single-pointed focus, you become aware of the mind's tendency to wander, while also strengthening your ability to intently stay with your point of concentration.

Dhyana

Dhyana is often referred to as "union." This is when concentration transforms into meditation. With long-held concentration, or dharana, the boundary between your sense of self as separate from the object upon which you are concentrating begins to dissolve.

Samadhi

Samadhi is considered the final stage of meditation: absorption with the supreme. Samadhi is an experience beyond description, and it is said it must be experienced to be known. We can think of this as the dissolution of the sense of self as separate from the whole, when duality falls away and a blissful state of union with the universe is experienced.

A Closing Note

This introduction to the practice and history of yoga is the smallest tip of the iceberg! I encourage you to continue to seek out other resources and guides and be mindful of what comes up for you physically, mentally, and emotionally as you explore your own yoga practice. Meet yourself with curiosity and compassion.

As you further your journey into this book and practice the asanas, listen to your body—it is your best teacher. There may be days or times of the day when some poses feel more accessible than others. Your variation of a pose does not have to be identical to the one you see in the book; you are a unique being with a unique background of experiences and your own individual anatomy. Although the written instructions for the poses include only one side, be sure to do any asymmetrical poses on both sides. Yoga is a practice of balance, after all. Be aware that, from one side to the other, things may feel different because we often have our own asymmetry when it comes to flexibility and strength. On top of that, former injuries may affect how you can move, so listen to your body and don't force anything that feels painful or unsafe. We hope this guide will serve you well on your journey into yoga, and we are so honored to walk this path with you, wherever you may be.

Collette Ouseley-Moynan

Desikachar, T.K.V. with R.H. Cravens. 2011. *Health, Healing, and Beyond: Yoga and the Living Tradition of T. Krishnamacharya*. New York: North Point Press.

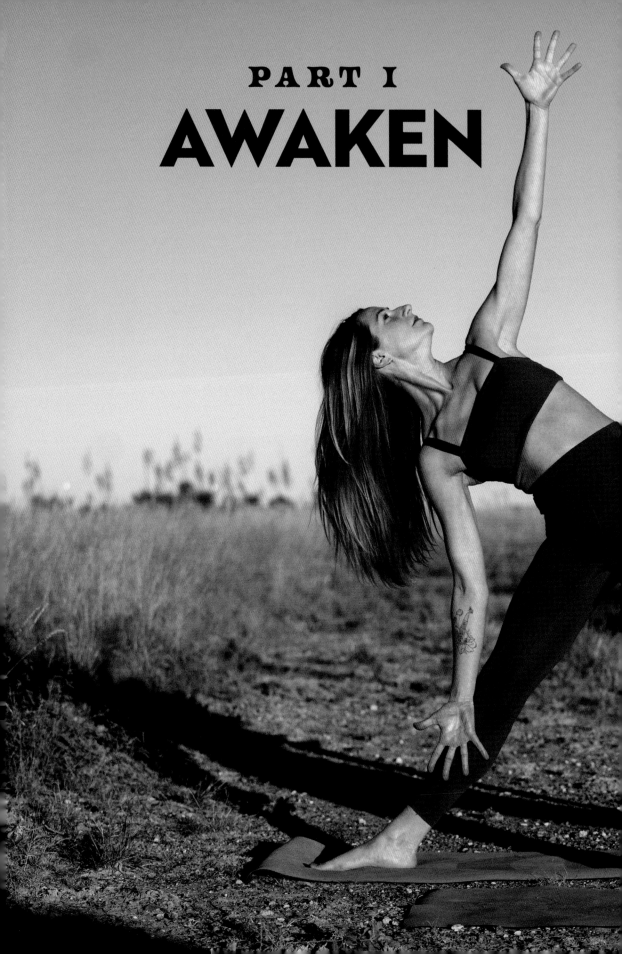

PART I
AWAKEN

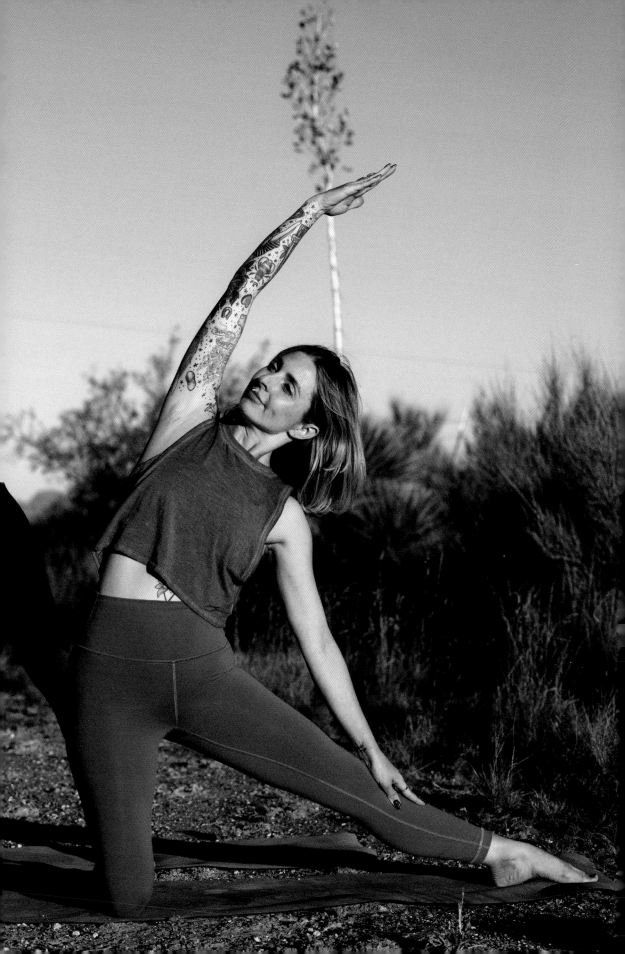

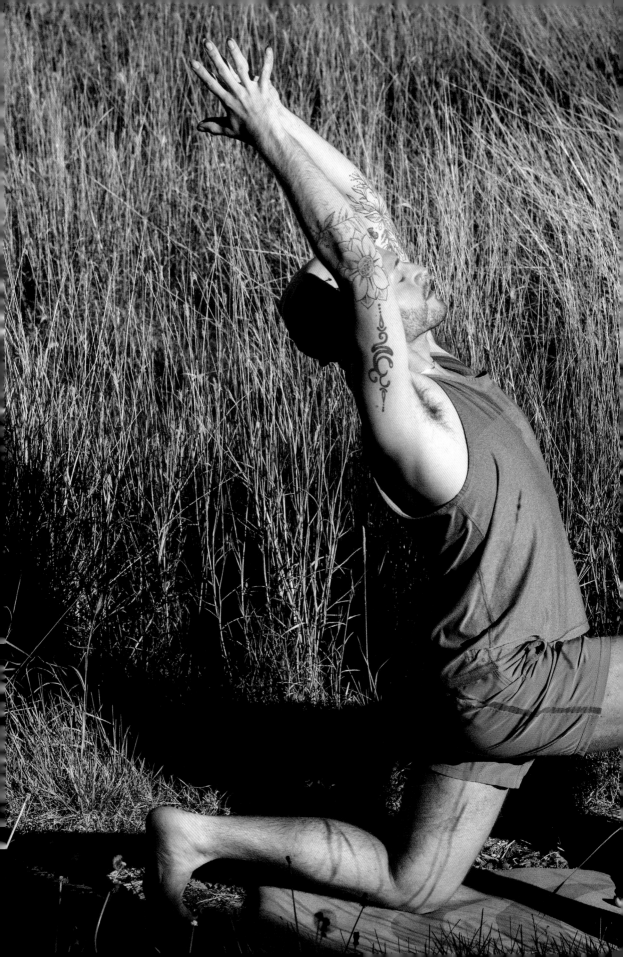

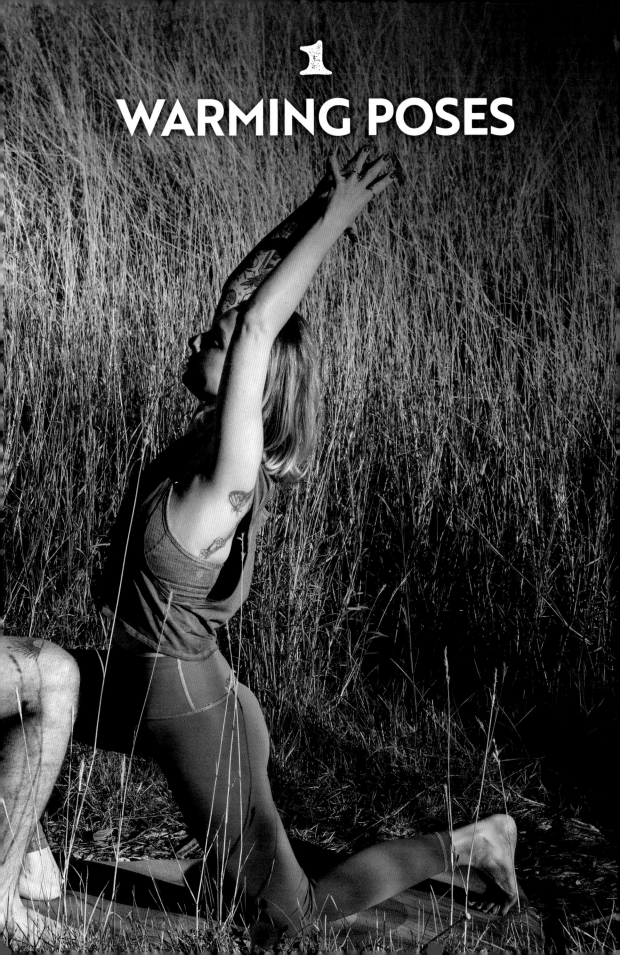

1
WARMING POSES

Mountain
Tadasana

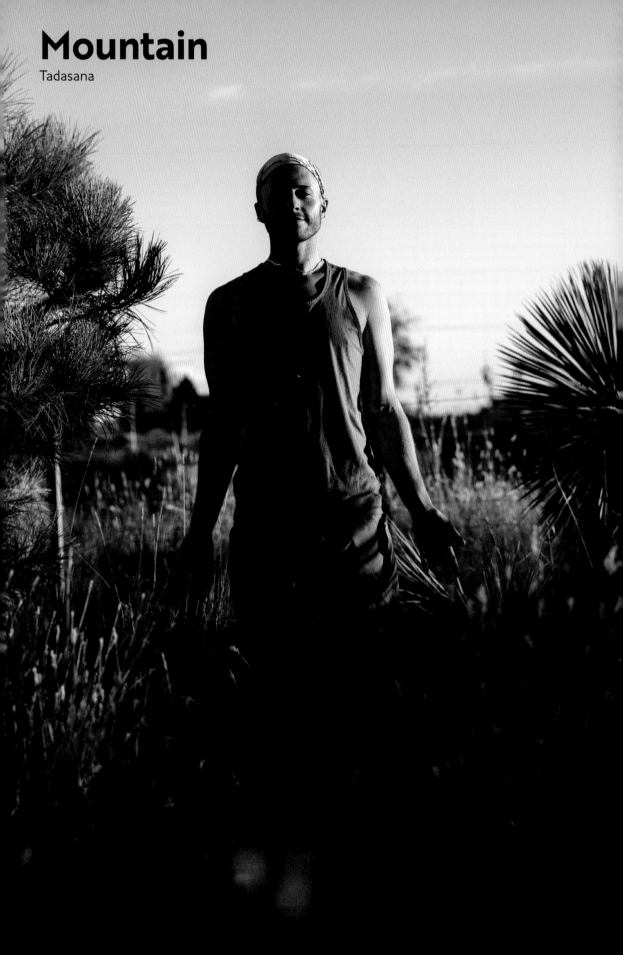

About This Pose

Mountain pose may not seem like a "pose" at first glance because it is a position we hold day in and day out. Its benefit is the opportunity to hold and experience this common position without being asked to do anything else. Becoming intimately aware of how you hold yourself in space is key for all your poses, and you can think of mountain pose as the blueprint for all other poses. A variation called upward salute or tall mountain (see first variation photo) is commonly used in a flow sequence on an inhale to create expansion and prepare for the next pose, such as forward fold in a sun salutation or another standing pose. The standing side bend, parsva tadasana (see second variation photo), adds a deep side bend to expand the rib cage while stretching and strengthening the core.

How To

- Stand with your feet roughly under your hip joints. This will most likely be a narrower stance than you anticipate. Aim to stack your hips over your knees and ankles so your thigh bones are vertical.
- Point all 10 toes forward so the outer edges of your feet are parallel to each other. Toes are in contact with the floor without gripping.
- Gently engage the pelvic floor muscles and deep core to lift your pubic bone so the pelvis is in a neutral position and shifted back over your heels and midfoot.
- Inhale, expanding the back and side ribs as you drop the bottom front ribs down to avoid rib flare.
- Relax your shoulders down away from your ears as you draw your shoulder blades inward toward the thoracic spine. For many people, this will feel like an opposing action to keeping the ribs down.
- Draw your ears slightly up and back, and bring your chin slightly in toward your neck to lengthen the cervical spine and bring your head in line over your shoulders.
- With a relaxed face and jaw, gaze forward or close your eyes to focus inward.

Variations

Upward Salute or Tall Mountain

From mountain pose, extend your arms overhead. Keep your arms as wide as your shoulders and wrap your biceps inward toward your ears. Keep your hands active while stretching your fingers upward.

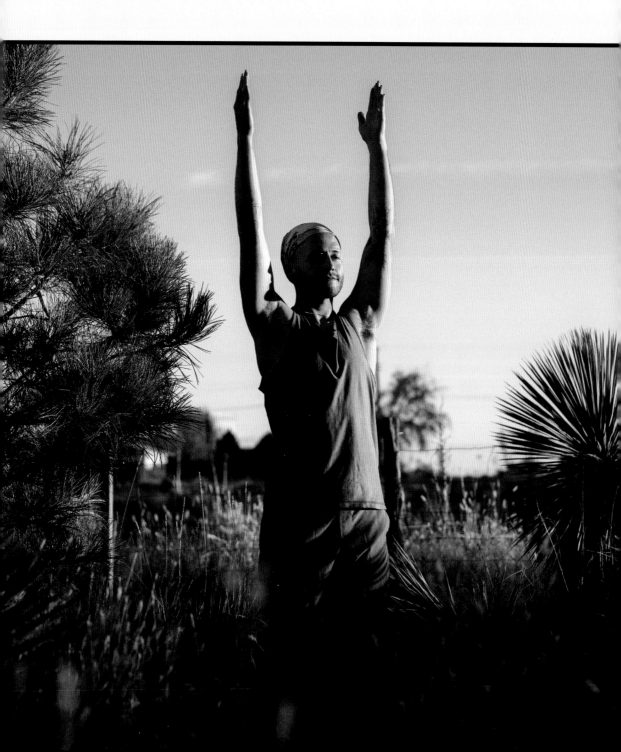

Standing Side Bend

With your arms extended above your head, interlace your fingers, but extend your index fingers upward. Press your palms together and draw your upper arms in toward your head as you inhale. As you exhale, press downward through your heels and the ball of each foot. Lean to the side, finding lateral flexion in your spine without collapsing the side of your body in the direction in which you are leaning. Use your bottom hand to gently pull on your top hand, bringing more length to the top arm.

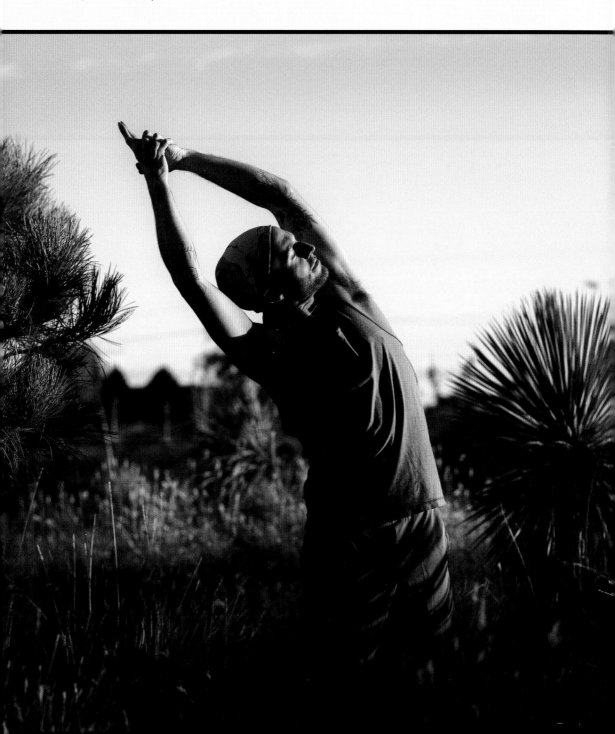

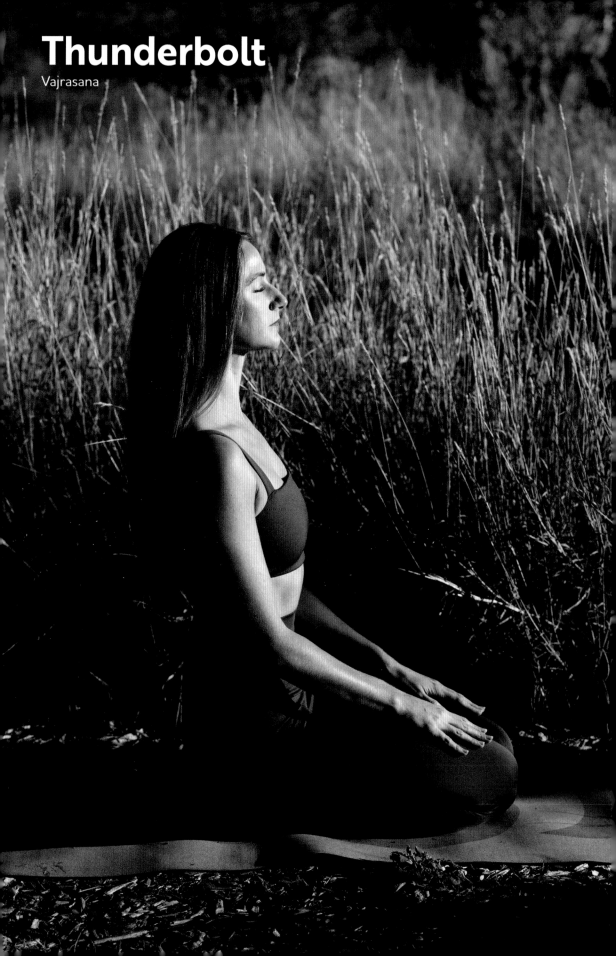

Thunderbolt
Vajrasana

About This Pose

Thunderbolt is a straightforward seated posture, but it is held for an extended period of time, which can be more challenging than you might expect. The pose stretches the front of your ankles and knees and allows space for diaphragmatic breathing, which in turn strengthens and relaxes the pelvic floor. Hero's pose, virasana, is a variation requiring more mobility in the lower legs. To make this pose more comfortable for your ankles, you may opt to use a thick blanket under your shins while your feet are on the ground.

How To

- Sit on your shins with the knees together and the feet a few inches apart.
- Shift your hips back toward your heels as far as you comfortably can without strain.
- Sit up tall and gently engage the lower core to lift the front of the pelvis and maintain a neutral position.
- Without flaring out your bottom ribs, relax the shoulder blades down your back.
- Gently pull your head up and back to lengthen the back of your neck.
- Focus your gaze on one point or close your eyes and observe the sensations inside your body and mind as you continue to sit (always without pain).

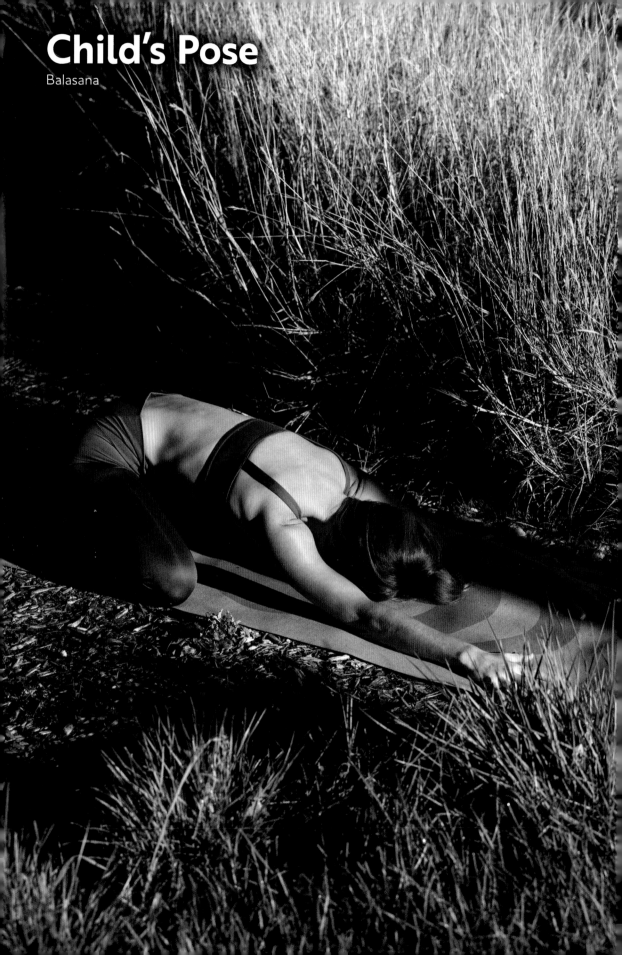

Child's Pose

Balasana

About This Pose

Child's pose is a kneeling posture that stretches the front of the ankles, quadriceps, lower back, and shoulders. Although it is commonly used as a resting pose in modern yoga practices, it still offers many benefits for your flexibility. A deep range of motion is required in your hips, knees, and ankles, and reaching your arms overhead can create a deep stretch in your lower back and latissimus muscles. It is a useful position to open space to be able to breath more fully into the back and sides of your lungs, increasing lung capacity. This pose also helps the body to prepare for more constricted poses.

How To

- From a tabletop position on your hands and knees, separate your knees wider than your hips.
- Shift your hips back toward your heels as far as you comfortably can without strain.
- Crawl forward with your hands as you relax your chest toward the floor. Separate your arms to shoulder-width apart or wider. Spread your fingers wide and place your hands fully on the ground.
- Inhale and expand the back and sides of your rib cage as you lengthen your spine.
- Exhale and engage the lower core as you relax to move your hips and chest closer to the floor.
- Rest your forehead on the mat and perhaps even roll your head side to side for a gentle neck release.

Lion's Pose

Simhasana

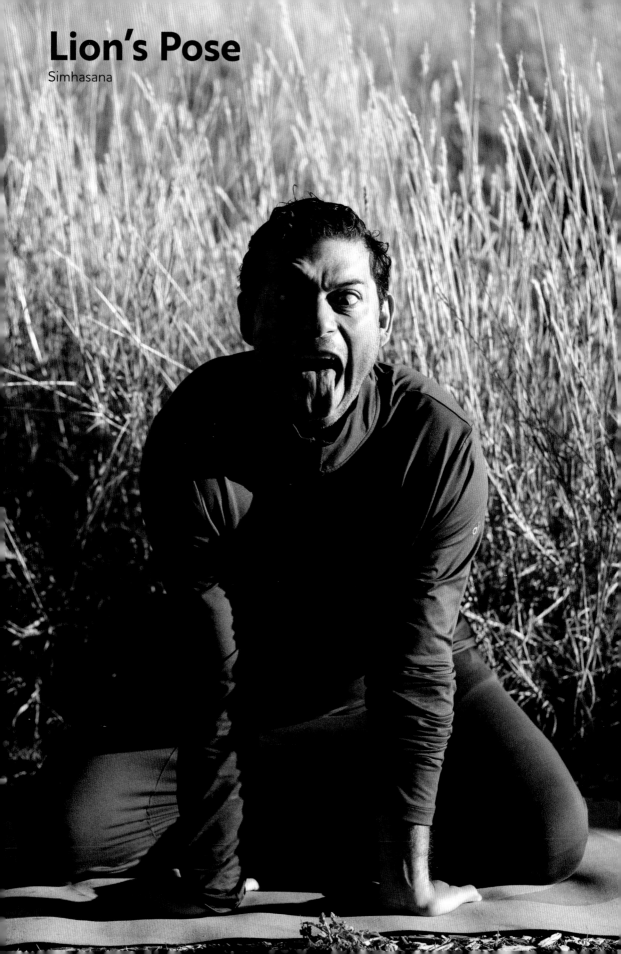

About This Pose

Lion's pose, or lion's breath, is a seated posture that uses forceful exhalations to wake up the body. It stretches the ankles and wrists while also relaxing the muscles of your face and throat. If you are practicing for the first time with others, it may feel awkward to make sounds, but that is part of the yoga practice as well!

How To

- From a seated position of vajrasana, separate your knees wide enough to place both hands on the mat between them with your palms flat. Turn your fingers toward your body.
- Inhale deeply to expand your rib cage on all sides.
- Extend your spine, and your gaze can be up to your forehead between your eyebrows.
- Stick out your tongue and exhale, making an audible "haaa" sound.
- Repeat four to six times.

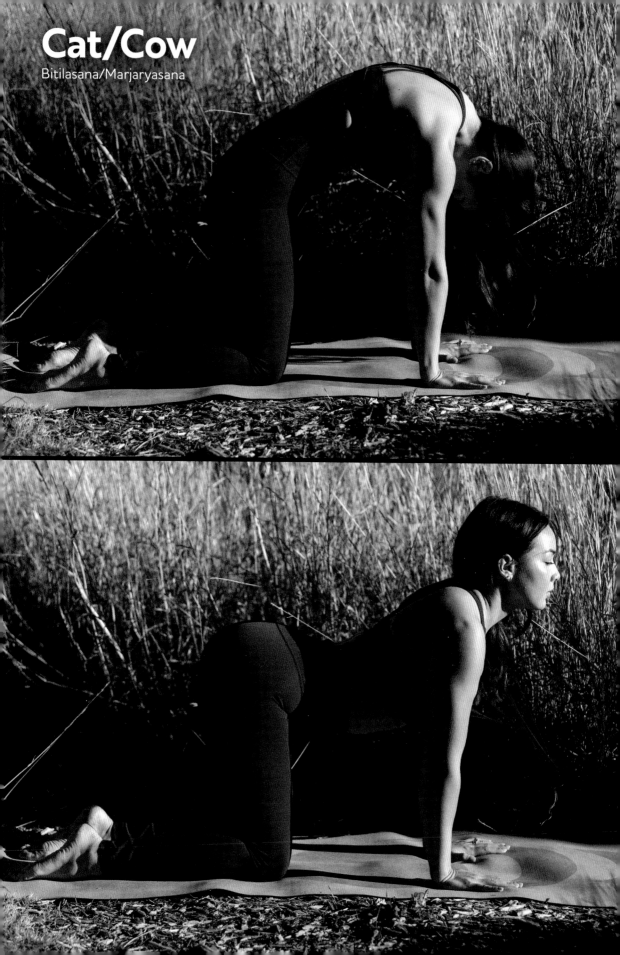

Cat/Cow
Bitilasana/Marjaryasana

About This Pose

No practice of mine can truly begin without multiple rounds of cat and cow—and usually several variations on the standard version. It is the perfect way to begin to warm up the spine as well as the wrist, shoulders, and hips. Take time to concentrate on how the two shapes and transitions feel in different areas of your body as you move. Cat pose engages the pectorals and abdominals, while cow uses the spinal extensors and latissimus. Feel free to play with different hand positions, and you can attempt to isolate the movement to parts of your spine (move only the pelvis, move only the rib cage, etc.).

How To

- Move into tabletop position: hands and knees with shoulders over your wrists and hips over your knees. Spread your fingers wide and press your knuckles firmly into the mat.
- For cat pose: Push the ground away with your hands and isometrically squeeze your hands toward one another. Tuck your chin to round your entire spine like an angry cat.

    - Isometrically squeeze your legs together to facilitate a deeper connection to your abdominals and tuck your tailbone.
    - Inhale into your back and side ribs.
    - Exhale to hollow out the lower belly and flex your spine more.

- For cow pose: Untuck your pelvis so your tailbone tilts upward. Energetically widen your thigh bones apart to engage the outer hip muscles and create more space to arch your lower back (spinal extension).

    - As you relax your rib cage toward the floor, drag your straightened arms toward your legs. This will engage your latissimus and draw the shoulders away from your ears, depressing the scapulae in and down the center spine.
    - If it is comfortable on your neck, lift your chin and gaze up at the center of your forehead.

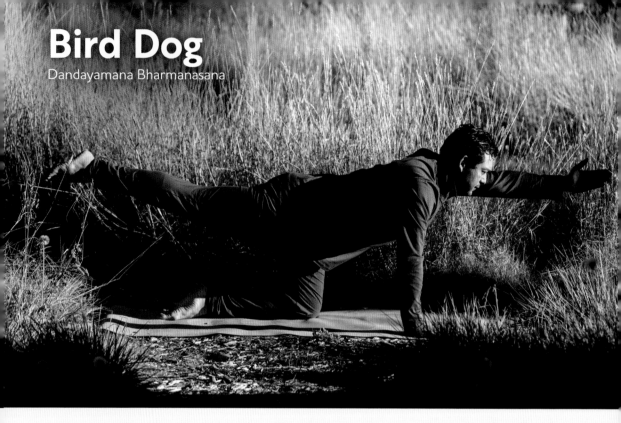

Bird Dog
Dandayamana Bharmanasana

About This Pose

This kneeling balance is an effective way to train the core for stability. Movement of the arms and legs, plus the force of gravity, increases the demand on the shoulders, core, and hips, so while it may look simple, this pose is not easy. If you have sensitive knees, use some extra padding for comfort. If your wrists are a concern, change the angle of your hands slightly or elevate the wrists higher than the knuckles and fingers so that you are on your fingertips (this will lessen the degree of extension needed). Many variations are possible—changing angles or adding movement can make the pose either more accessible or more difficult.

How To

- From tabletop, engage the core to keep your spine and pelvis in a neutral position. Gaze at the floor between your hands.
- Extend one leg straight behind you. Point or flex the foot—imagine pulling your toes toward your nose—and push out through your heel so the leg is strong and straight.
- Push your hands into the floor to activate your chest and front shoulder muscles. This action brings your shoulder blades toward your side ribs and lifts your upper thoracic spine toward the ceiling.
- Reach your opposite arm forward, with your upper arm by your ear and your thumb pointed upward.
- Keep the spine and hips still as you inhale and stretch in opposite directions.
- Exhale to connect to your deep core and squeeze the glutes to keep your leg lifted.
- Hold for the desired number of breaths, then repeat on the other side.

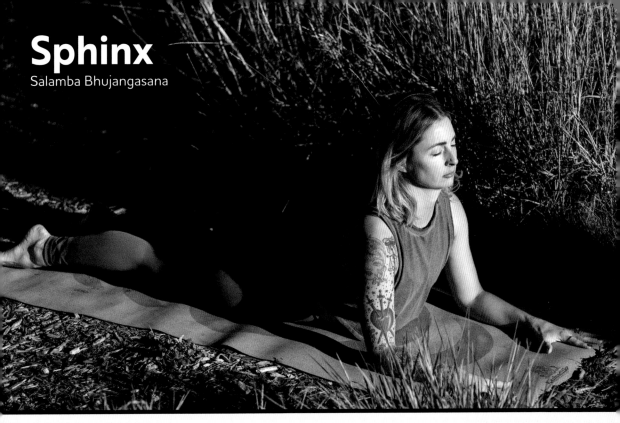

Sphinx
Salamba Bhujangasana

About This Pose

As an invitation into upper and middle back extension, sphinx can be a gentle, sustainable introductory backbend on your journey. Yin yoga teaches a fully passive, relaxed variation, but as a warming pose for a full hatha practice, here you activate the legs, core, and back muscles to wake up the body and prepare for deeper backbends.

How To

- Lying face down on your mat, prop your elbows underneath your shoulders. Separate the forearms so they are roughly parallel, like the number "11."
- Engage your leg muscles as you push the tops of your feet into the floor and activate the glutes. Draw the lower core in to stabilize your pelvis and provide length to the lumbar spine.
- Press your elbows, forearms, and hands into the ground and simultaneously retract the shoulder blades together on your back to open the chest.
- Play with shifting your gaze forward, down, or up without strain to stretch various parts of your neck.

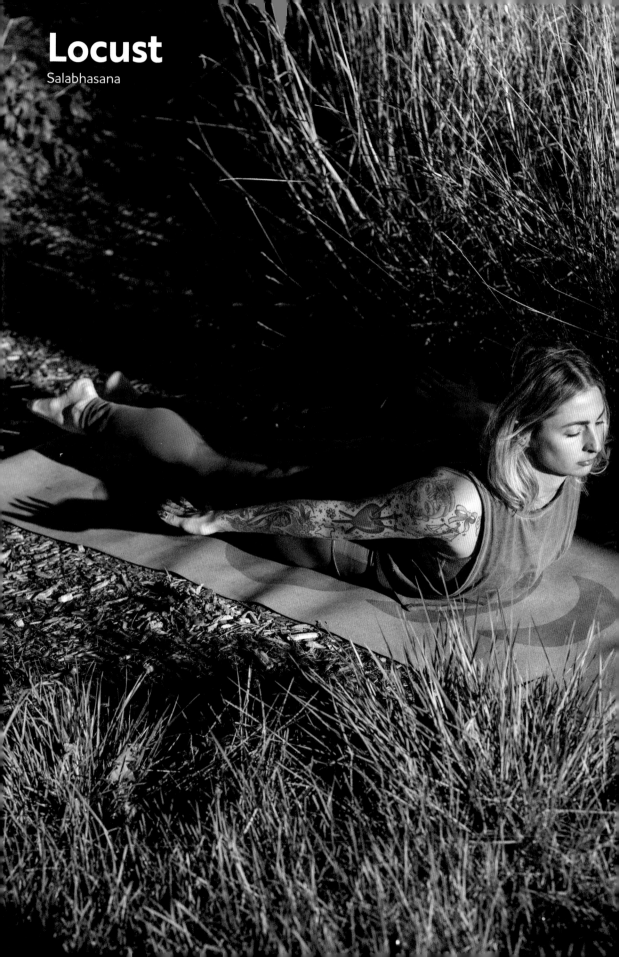

Locust
Salabhasana

About This Pose

Locust builds strength in the entire posterior chain as you lift yourself up against gravity. As you lift, be mindful that the lower back muscles will typically try to do most of the work because spinal extension is their primary job. Use the muscles along the entire length of your spine and the back of your hips and legs not only to lift higher but also to create a stronger, more sustainable shape.

How To

- Lying face down on the mat, stretch your arms close by your sides, with palms facing down.
- Draw your shoulder blades together on your back (retraction) and reach for your toes to depress the scapulae and engage your latissimus muscles.
- Hug your leg muscles tight and point your toes.
- Inhale, expand your rib cage on all sides, and lengthen your spine.
- Exhale and activate all the muscles in the back of your body to lift both your legs and your torso away from the floor.
- Look down and slightly draw your chin inward before gently lifting your head.
- Experiment with arm variations out to the sides, like a "T," or overhead for different sensations in your mid and upper back muscles.

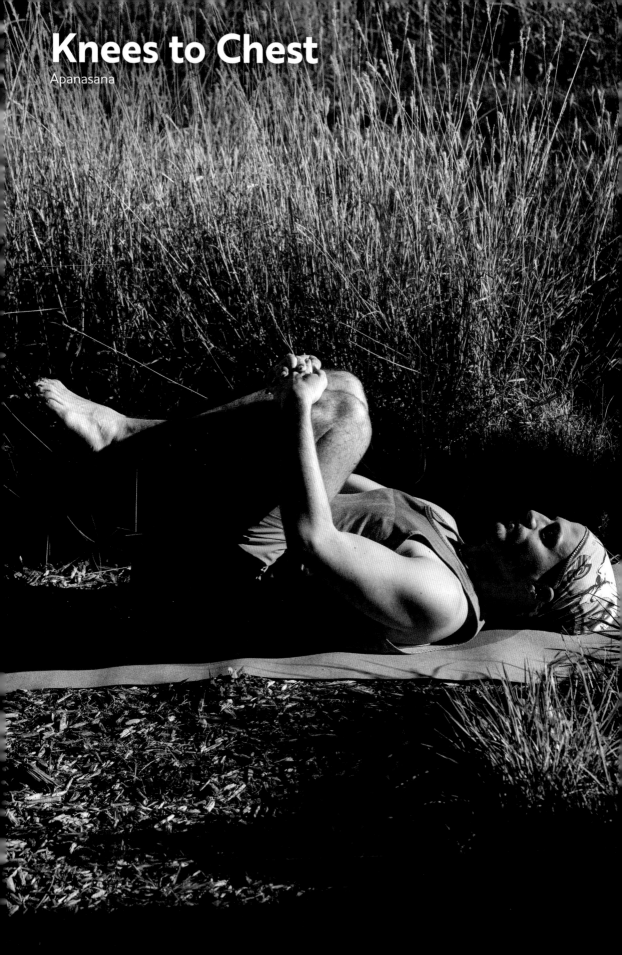

Knees to Chest

Apanasana

About This Pose

Apanasana can be a wonderful way to relax the lower back and gently stretch the hips and upper hamstrings. Because it is a reclined pose, there is much less effort required compared with standing poses, and gravity can aid you as you relax into the shape. Add some movement by making small circles with your knees to massage the lower back.

How To

- Lie down with your legs stretched out on the floor and arms by your sides.
- On an exhale, engage the lower core and draw both knees into your chest. Clasp the front of your shins with your hands or grab opposite elbows if your arms allow.
- Keep your head relaxed on the floor, with your chin slightly tucked. If needed, a block or pillow under your head is a nice support.
- To see what your hips prefer, try keeping your pelvis rooted to the floor and allowing it to lift.

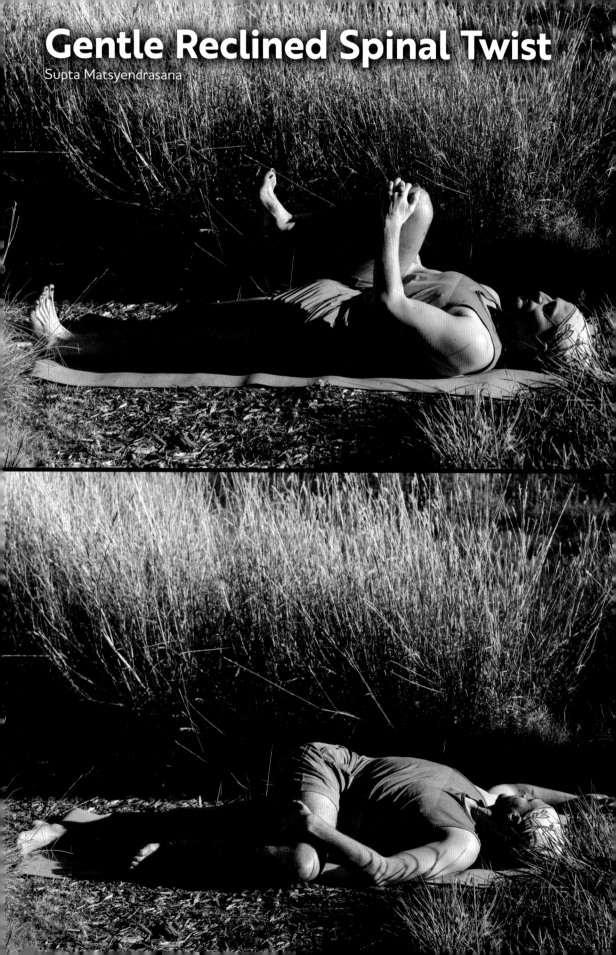

Gentle Reclined Spinal Twist
Supta Matsyendrasana

About This Pose

Twists can be used as a way to clear out stagnation and fatigue, and they are also vital to include in yoga practice because most modern movement is linear—forward and backward. This pose can be included in a warm-up or cool-down sequence.

How To

- Lie down with your legs extended out on the floor and your arms by your sides.
- On an exhale, engage the lower core and hug one knee into your chest.
- Cross your knee to the opposite side until your hips are stacked.
- Extend your opposite arm out and turn your rib cage back toward the floor.
- Gaze up at the ceiling, keeping your neck straight and neutral, or turn to look past your extended hand.
- Inhale to expand the back and side of your rib cage.
- Exhale to activate the obliques to deepen the twist.

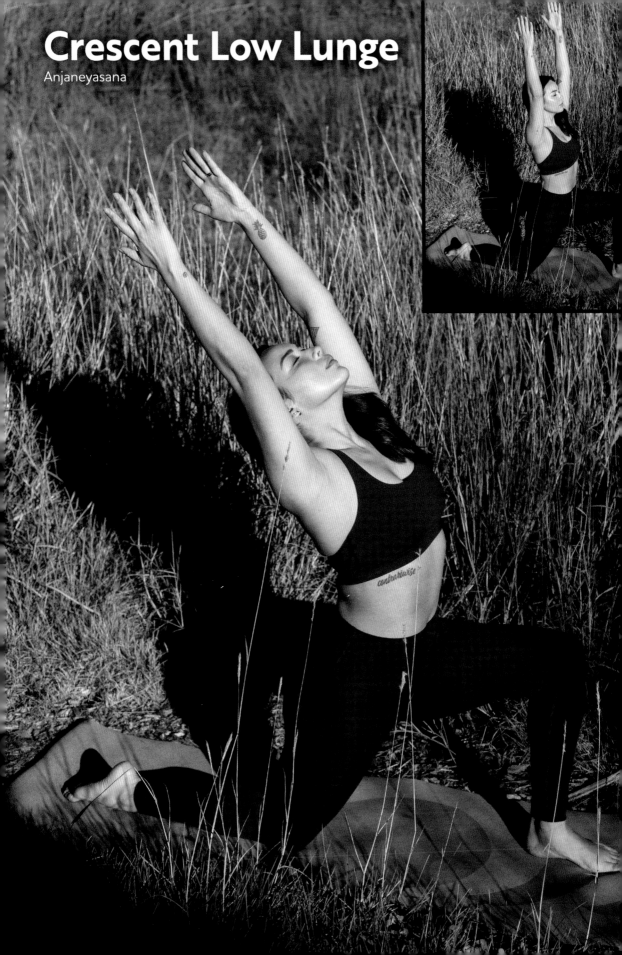

Crescent Low Lunge
Anjaneyasana

About This Pose

Crescent low lunge stretches the hip flexors while activating the glutes and hamstrings. Variations add a backbend and abdominal stretch, which can be beneficial for stronger standing poses. Crescent low lunge is also a great pose for maintaining good posture and creating mobility for lower-body strength training.

How To

- From a standing forward fold, step one foot back and lower your knee to the ground. Tuck or untuck your toes, depending on your own comfort and mobility.
- Inhale and lift your torso upright as you bring your arms overhead.
- Squeeze your glutes and activate your deep core to lift your pubic bone up and drop your tailbone down. The more you lunge forward, the more challenging this work becomes, so pull back as needed to position your pelvis upright.
- Stretch your rib cage up away from your hips and gently bend back. The more you coil up, the more space you create to bend back.
- Look down and slightly draw your chin in toward your neck before looking up to maintain length in the back of the neck to prevent strain.

Crescent Low Lunge Twist

Parivrtta Anjaneyasana

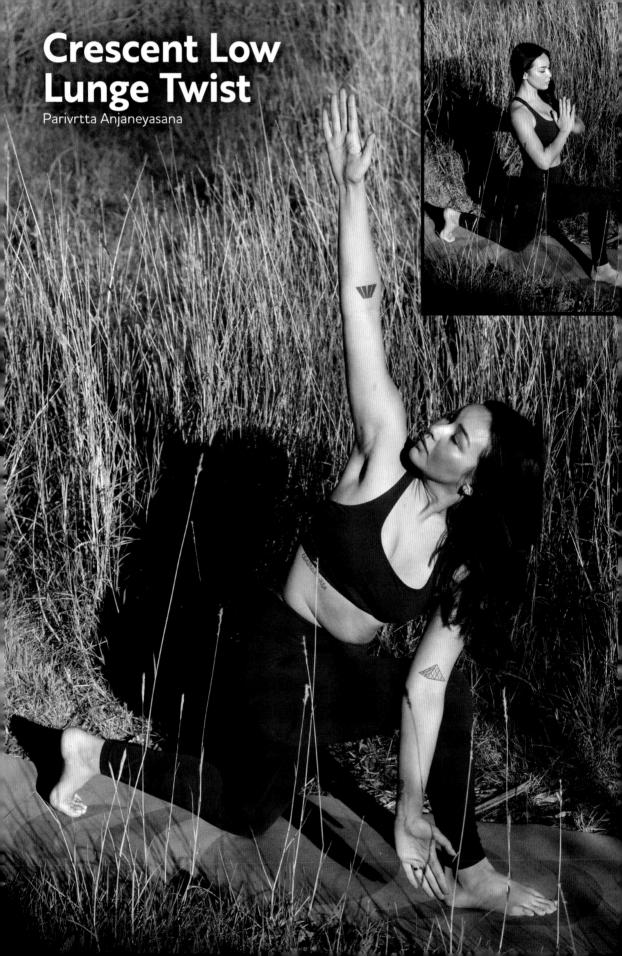

About This Pose

This pose takes the base of a low lunge and adds in a spinal twist. Twists are essential in training for common lifestyle movements, and this pose offers an opportunity to twist with a lesser likelihood of revolving in the pelvis because the back knee is on the floor and helps to stabilize the lower body. Crescent low lunge twist stretches the glutes of the front leg, hip flexors of the back leg, and the chest, while also strengthening the core.

How To

- From a forward fold, move your left foot to the back of your mat, lower the left knee, and bring both hands to the floor. The front foot and back knee are roughly hip-width apart. The toes of the back foot can be tucked or untucked.
- With your front knee over your heel, push down into the floor with your foot to engage the entire leg and hip.
- Energetically hug your legs toward one another to stabilize your lower body. Place your right hand on your front thigh as you extend your left arm to the ceiling.
- Rotate your rib cage toward your front leg, hook your left arm on the outer right thigh, and bring your hands together palm to palm.
- Continue to breathe and engage your core as you twist incrementally toward your front leg with each exhale.
- Option (pictured): Open your arms with your top right hand aligned over the right shoulder and your left arm still hooked to the outside of your front leg, with the left hand near the outer ankle of your front foot. Gaze in the direction of your chest or look up past your top hand if it is comfortable for your neck.

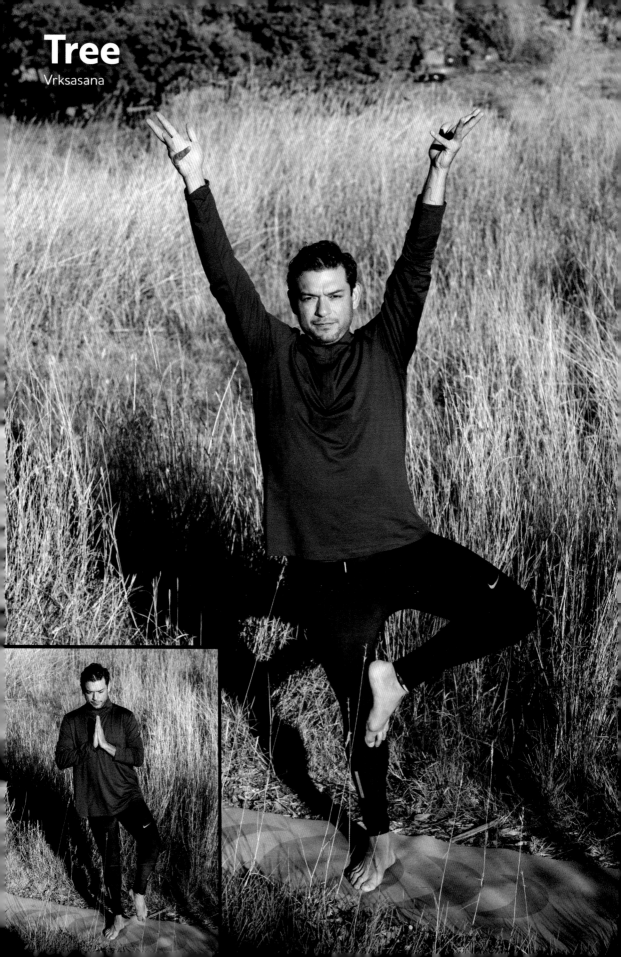

Tree
Vrksasana

About This Pose

Tree pose is a foundational, one-leg standing pose combining strength, stability, balance, and focus. It requires strength in the standing leg, outer hip of the lifted leg, and deep core. While you engage and pull your core in to find stability, at the same time, you must lengthen the spine in axial extension, reaching your tailbone toward the floor while simultaneously lengthening through the neck, reaching the crown of your head up toward the sky.

How To

- From mountain pose, shift your weight more to one leg and lift your opposite foot off the floor.
- Place your lifted foot on your standing leg's inner thigh or to the inside of the lower leg. Press your foot into your standing leg while pushing your standing leg back against your foot.
- Lift up through the deep core and activate the outer hip of your lifted leg to open the knee externally, thus creating a stretch on the inner thigh. While the thigh bone rotates externally, do not turn in the pelvis; keep your hip bones squared off to the front of your mat.
- Rest your hands together at your heart or reach your arms overhead.
- Gaze down at a point in front of you, look up, or for even more of a balance challenge, close your eyes.

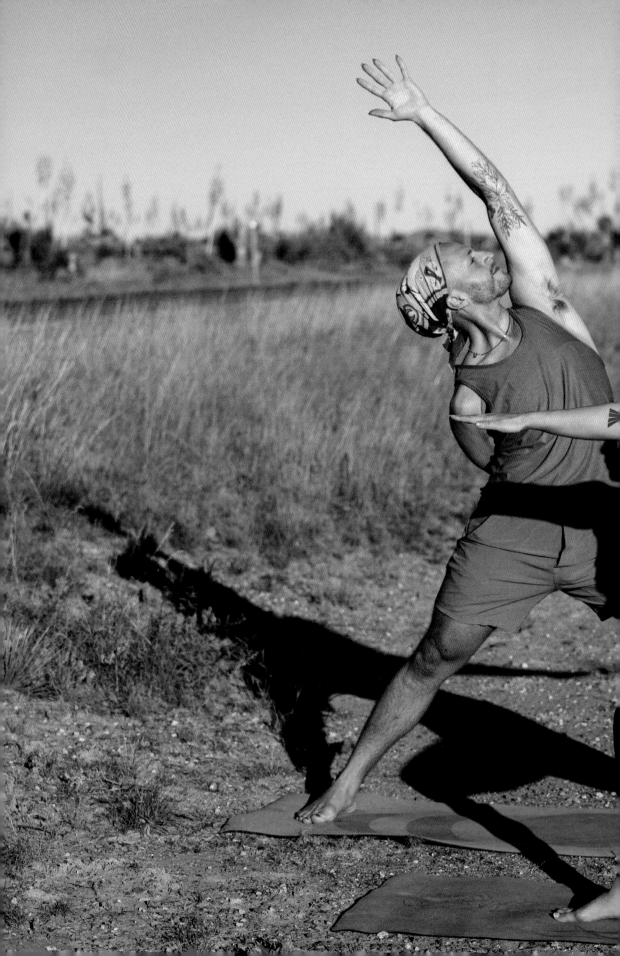

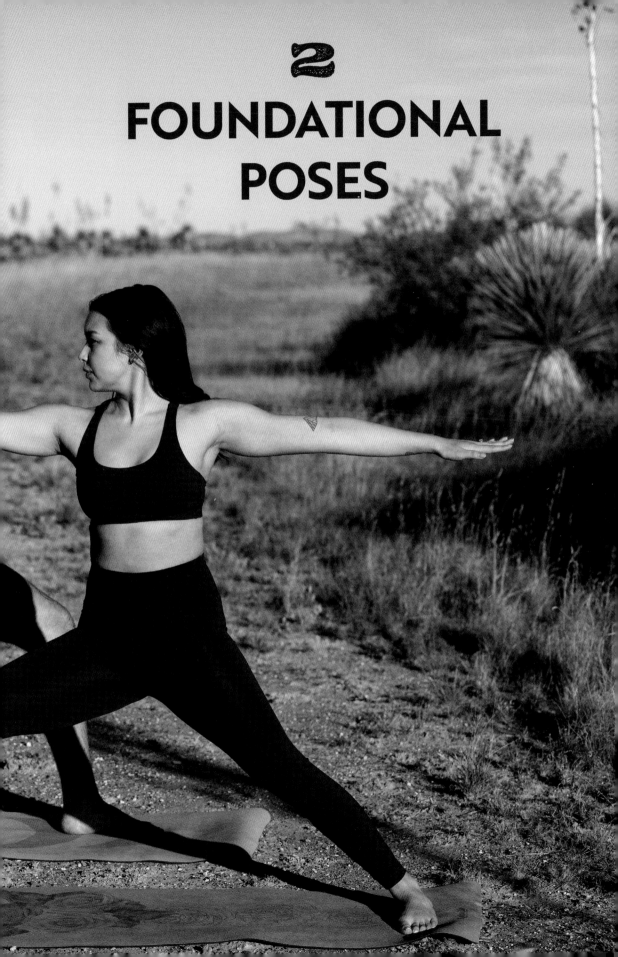

2
FOUNDATIONAL POSES

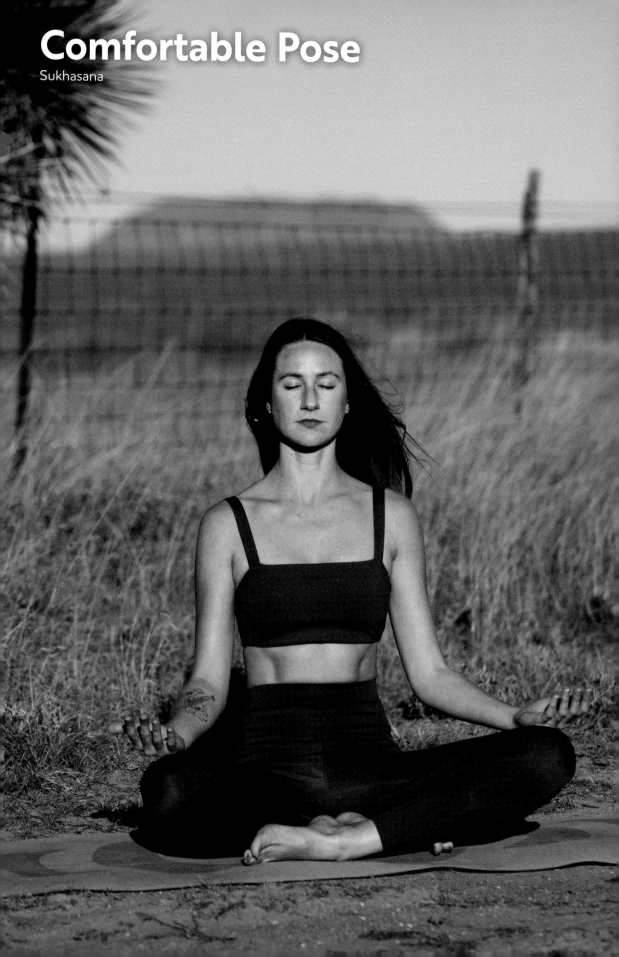

Comfortable Pose
Sukhasana

About This Pose

Comfortable pose definitely requires effort, especially because most of us don't very often sit up tall without a support behind us. It may take time to build up the endurance to maintain this pose for an extended amount of time, but this posture is great for meditation and pranayama. Feel free to also add in movements such as cat and cow, twists (see variation photo), or side bends as a warm-up for your hips and spine.

How To

- Sit on the floor with your pelvis upright and neutral.
- Cross your shins in front of your pelvis. If your knees are elevated above your hips, elevate your hips by sitting on a folded blanket, pillow, or bolster.
- Rest your hands on your legs, palms down—or in your lap with palms up.
- Inhale and lengthen your entire spine up through the crown of your head.
- Exhale to bring the lower belly in and up as you keep the shoulders relaxed down and back.
- Gaze softly out in front of you or close your eyes.

Variation

Comfortable Pose With Spinal Twist

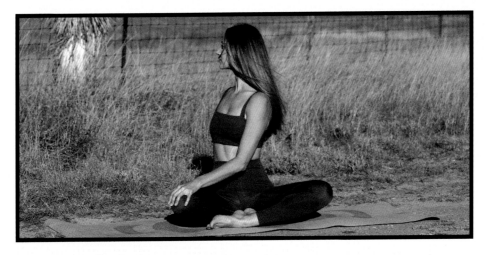

From comfortable pose, inhale and reach your arms overhead, biceps turned inward toward your ears. Exhale, turn to the right, place the fingertips of your right hand behind you on the floor, and place your left hand on your right leg. Inhale to lengthen the spine like you are reaching the top of your head to the sky and rooting your tailbone into the ground at the same time. Exhale to deepen the twist leading from your core. Keep your shoulder blades pulled together at the spine to maintain an open chest. Relax the shoulders and look over your back shoulder. Switch sides.

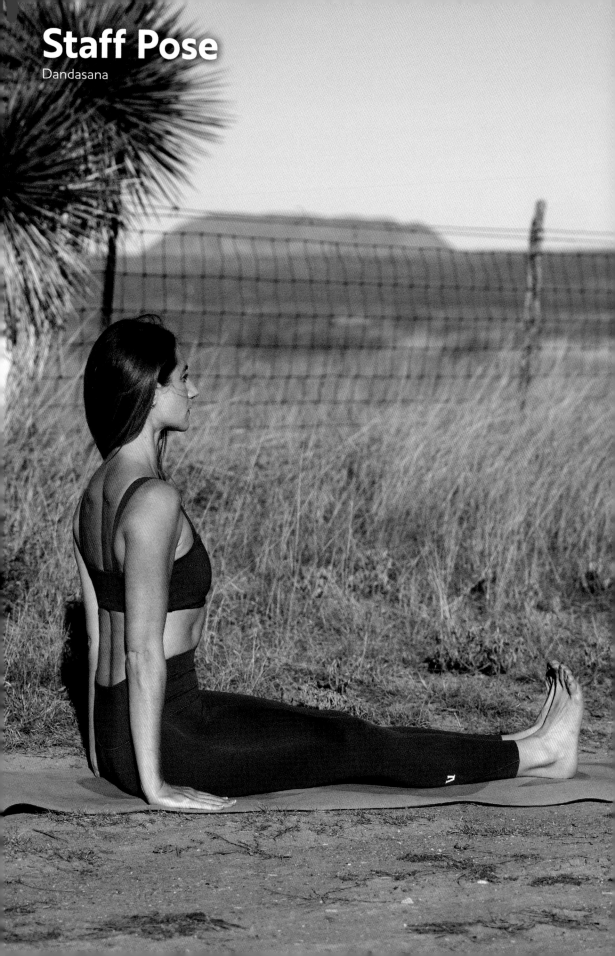

Staff Pose

Dandasana

About This Pose

Staff pose is a straightforward seated posture that offers subtle but powerful benefits. You will strengthen your core and back extensors to sit up tall, as well as stretch the back of your legs and feet by engaging the muscles on the front of your legs. The longer you stay—and the more restricted the mobility in your hips—the more challenging it will be to remain upright, so take your time to build endurance in this pose.

How To

- Sit on the floor with your legs stretched out in front of you. The legs may be glued together or separated to hip-distance apart. Elevate your hips on a pillow or blanket to make this more accessible and comfortable.
- Flex your ankles to bring the tops of your feet toward your face and squeeze the quadriceps to tighten your knees.
- Without tilting your pelvis too far forward or backward, bring your lower belly in and up as you anchor your hips into the floor.
- Keep the bottom front ribs down as you move your shoulder blades back to open your chest.
- Press your palms into the floor next to your hips and actively sink your shoulders toward the floor to engage your latissimus muscles. If your arms are long relative to your spine, you can elevate your hips. If your arms seem too short and you can't press your palms flat, roll the tops of the shoulders back and down while drawing the shoulder blades inward toward your spine.
- Slightly tuck your chin and gaze forward or close your eyes.

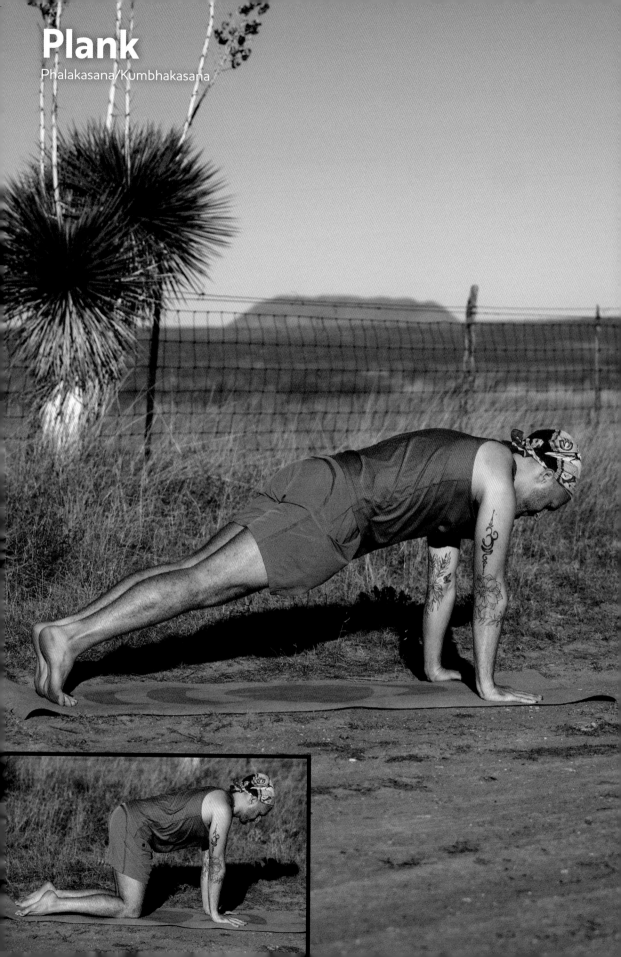

Plank
Phalakasana/Kumbhakasana

About This Pose

Plank is an integral part of the modern sun salutation. While the emphasis may be on upper-body strength, plank is a full-body pose that also works the legs and core. A common variation that reduces the demands on your wrists but can feel more challenging for your core is forearm plank (see variation photo).

How To

- In a tabletop position on your hands and knees, align your shoulders over your hands. Spread all 10 fingers wide as you press your knuckles and finger pads into the mat and hold.
- Push the ground away to elevate the upper back between your shoulder blades, like a hint of cat pose. Isometrically squeeze your thumbs toward one another to build more strength in the chest, serratus, and biceps.
- Engage the deep core to stabilize the pelvis and keep it from sinking toward the floor.
- One at a time, extend your legs out behind you—either hip-width apart or squeezed together.
- Press your heels into an imaginary wall at the back of your mat to engage the glutes and legs. At the same time, extend the crown of your head in the opposite direction.
- Gaze at the floor between your fingers.

Variation

Forearm Plank

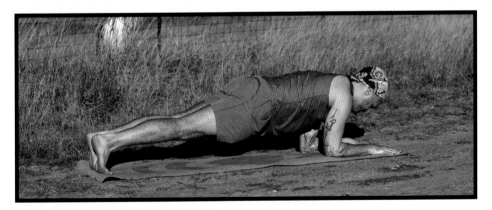

From tabletop, place your forearms on the floor, align your elbows under your shoulders, and keep your forearms parallel to one another, palms face down. Push the ground down with your forearms to elevate the upper back between your shoulder blades, as in plank. Isometrically squeeze your forearms together without your elbows splaying wider than your shoulders. Engage the deep core to stabilize the pelvis and keep it from sinking to the floor. One at a time, walk your feet back behind you, keeping the legs either hip-width apart or with feet together. On tiptoes, press your heels into an imaginary wall at the back of your mat to engage the glutes and legs. At the same time, extend the crown of your head forward, gazing on the ground to keep the neck long.

Four-Limb Staff

Chaturanga Dandasana

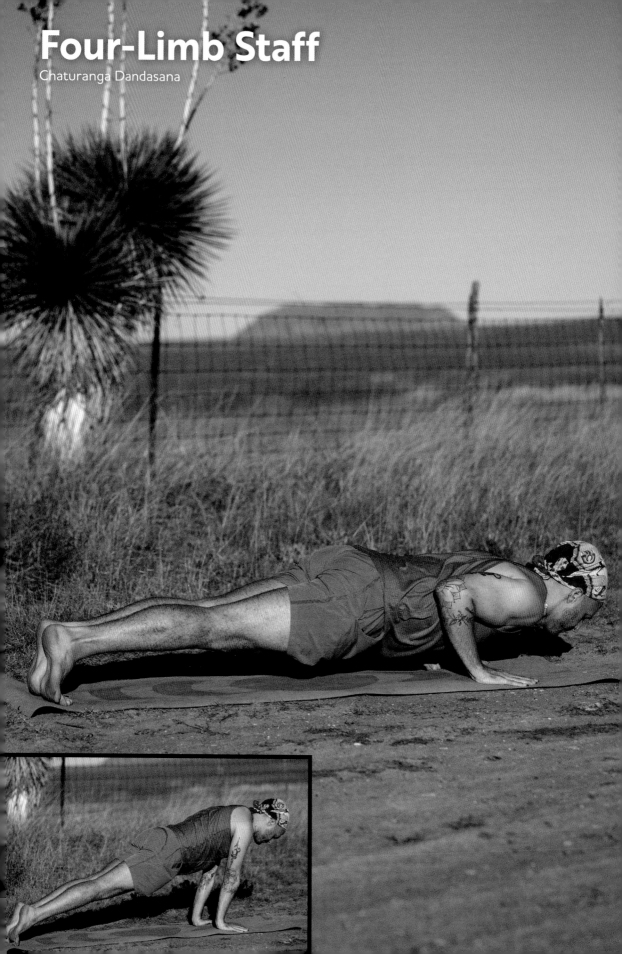

About This Pose

Chaturanga dandasana is an integral part of the modern sun salutation as you transition into upward-facing dog or cobra. Like plank, four-limb staff may feel like a purely upper-body strengthener—you are essentially holding the bottom of a push-up—but it requires stability in the legs and core to be both effective and safe. To spend more time in the pose and build strength, an effective variation is to lower your knees so the load in your upper body is manageable but still challenging.

How To

- From plank pose, keep your legs and core strong and stiff as a board. Move yourself slightly forward so your shoulders are past your wrists.
- Bend your elbows to lower your shoulders toward the floor until they are roughly the same height as your elbows. Elbows are close to the ribs but not so much that they are supporting the weight of your rib cage.
- Push your hands down into the floor to engage the serratus and stabilize the shoulder blades.
- Keep your neck long as you gaze at the floor.

Side Plank
Vasisthasana

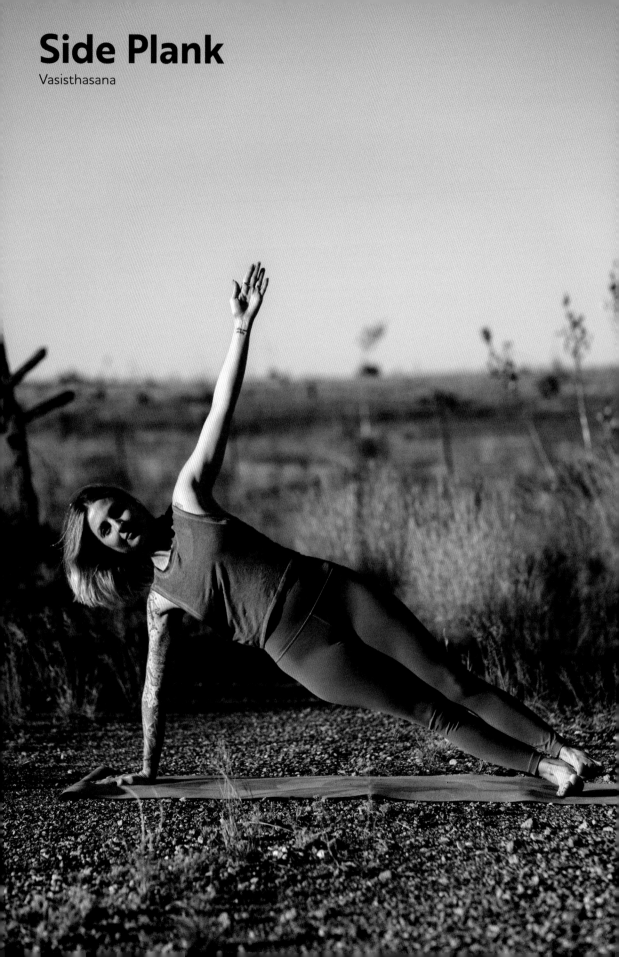

About This Pose

Side plank takes the standard plank with two hands and adds a balance challenge. It requires strength in the entire body—especially in the obliques on the sides of your waist. Many variations on this pose introduce different sensations of strength and stretch. My favorite adds a hip flexor and outer hip stretch for the top thigh while adding more support and taking some load off the bottom arm (see variation photo).

How To

- From plank pose, pivot your feet to one side so that your feet are stacked one ankle on top of the other, then balance on the outer edge of your bottom foot. Energize your feet by flexing them and spread your toes to prevent rolling toward the top of your foot while you push the edge of your bottom foot into the ground.
- Extend your top arm straight upward above the top shoulder as you simultaneously push your opposite hand into the floor beneath your bottom shoulder. The hips and chest will face the side of your space.
- Engage the outer hip muscles and obliques on the bottom of your waist to keep your pelvis lifted away from the floor.
- Gaze forward or up past your top hand.

Variation

Supported Side Plank With Hip Opener

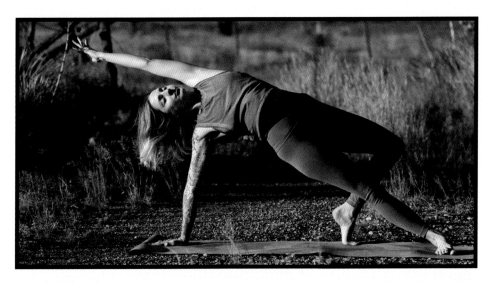

From side plank, put your top leg behind your bottom leg and bend the top knee to place the tiptoes of the top foot on the ground behind your bottom thigh or knee. Continue to press down through your bottom hand while reaching up through your top arm and hand. Keep the front of your body facing the side of your space and lift your top hip upward to create a stretch for the top outer hip and a slight side bend along your torso.

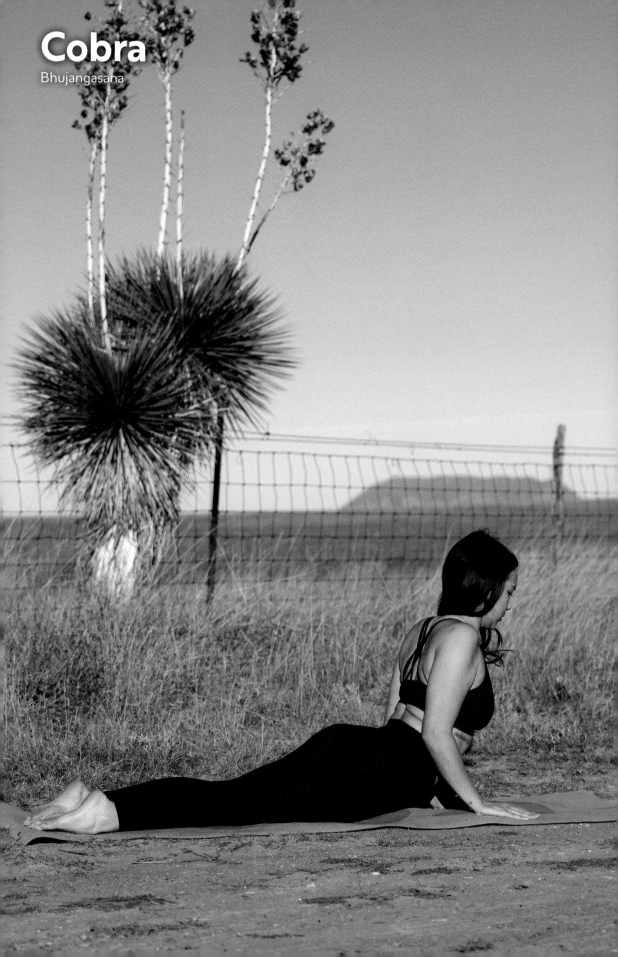

Cobra
Bhujangasana

About This Pose

Cobra is a foundational backbend that strengthens the back and legs while stretching the front of the body. It is often used as an alternative to upward-facing dog in the sun salutation; however, it is a wonderful backbend for all yogis to incorporate. This backbend focuses on strengthening the back extensors without the requirement of balancing on your hands. To build even more strength, once you are lifted, try to lift your hands and hover them above the floor by the sides of your rib cage.

How To

- Lying face down on the floor, press your palms flat beside your ribs.
- Press the tops of your feet into the ground so your legs are strong. Engage the lower core to stabilize your pelvis.
- Squeeze your shoulder blades together (retraction) and toward your hips (depression) to expand your chest.
- Inhale—expanding your rib cage on all sides as you lengthen your spine away from your hips.
- Exhale—keeping the lower belly engaged as you coil your chest up away from the floor.
- You can gaze forward or gently lift your chin and look up. Avoid forcing your head back. Continuously coil your chest forward and up to increase the thoracic extension.

Boat
Navasana

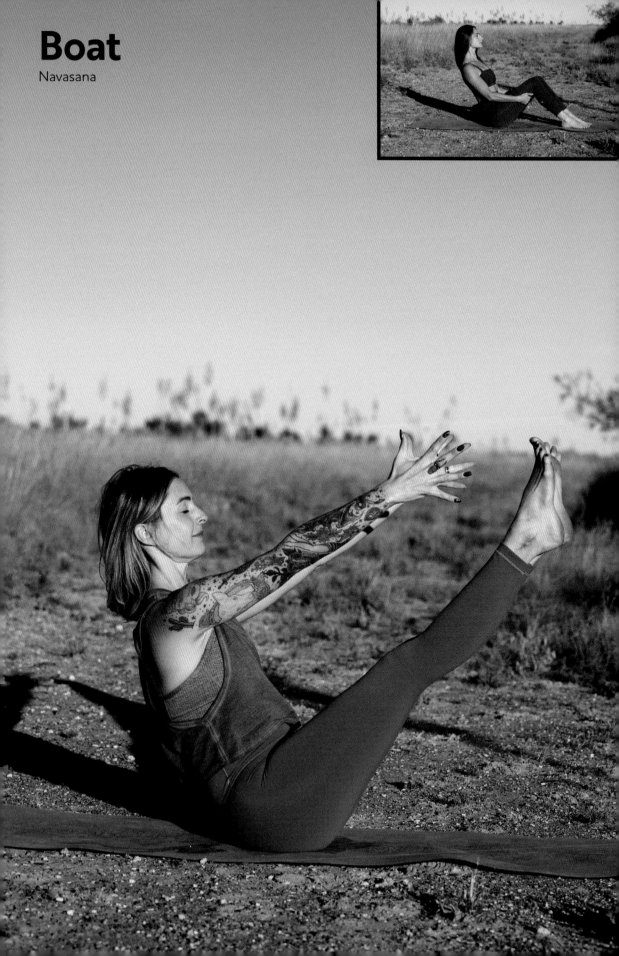

About This Pose

Boat is a seated pose that specifically targets the abdominals and hip flexors, but it also requires strength in the legs and back. From this pose, you can incorporate different shapes in the upper body and legs. The variation I sequence most often for inversion prep is the low boat (see variation photo).

How To

- From a seated position with your legs in front of you, bend your knees and press your feet into the floor. Lightly support the backs of your knees with your hands and sit up tall.
- Drop your shoulders down away from your ears without arching the upper back so the rib cage stays in a neutral position.
- Tuck your pelvis slightly and rock backward until you balance on your sitz bones and your feet lift off the floor.
- Tighten the deep core between your hip bones and above your pubic bone.
- If this is going well, squeeze your quadriceps to extend both legs and reach your arms forward.

Variation

Low Boat

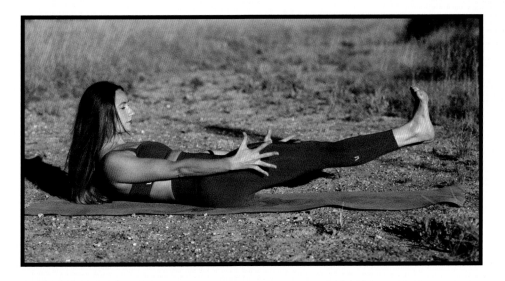

From boat pose, lower your legs and torso as low to the floor as possible while keeping your deep core engaged. Draw your navel inward toward your spine to keep a bowl-like shape, curving inward at your center. If your lower back arches away from the ground, lift your legs higher.

Reverse Tabletop

Ardha Purvottanasana

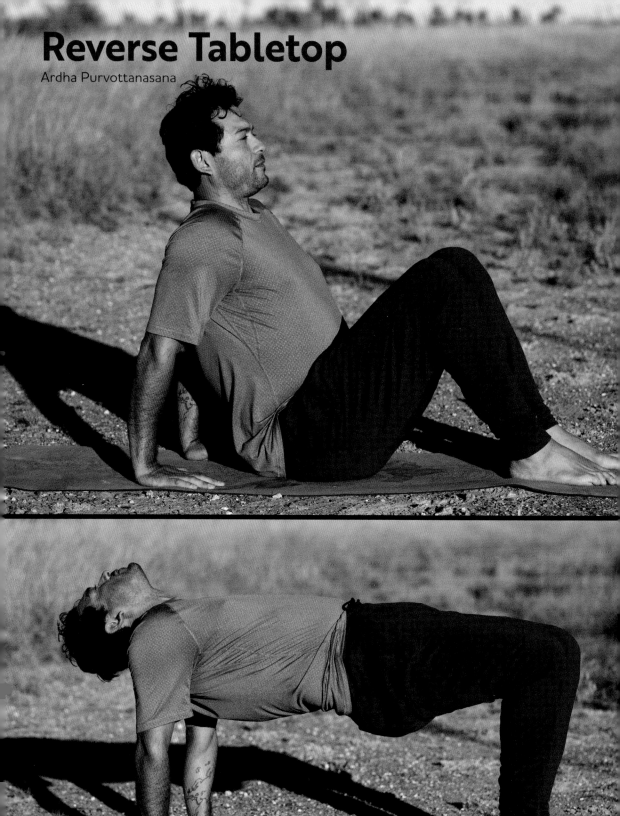

About This Pose

Sometimes called crab, this foundational pose builds strength and endurance in the posterior chain. It also strengthens the shoulders in extension and internal rotation, which is an action that relatively few other poses require. Reverse plank (see variation photo) is a progression of this pose, with higher demand on the deep core and glutes when legs are straight.

How To

- From a seated position, lean your upper body back and place your hands on the floor behind you. Fingers turned toward you will be the highest demand on your wrists, so find an angle with fingers turned to the sides or even to the back that is comfortable and stable.
- Bend your knees and place your feet hip-distance apart.
- Inhale and push your hands into the floor to engage the upper back and arms and open the chest.
- Exhale as you squeeze your glutes and push your feet down to lift your hips high.
- Engage the deep core and the glutes to keep your pelvis and lumbar spine neutral. This will stretch the hip flexors and thighs.
- Continue to push through your hands and contract the upper back muscles to open the chest.
- If it is comfortable on your neck, gently drop your head back.

Variation

Reverse Plank

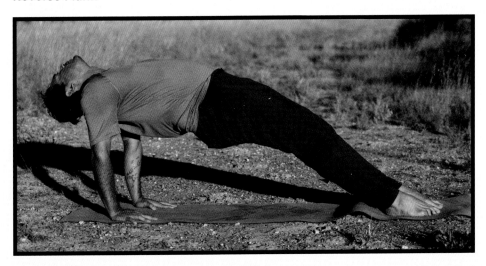

From reverse tabletop, continue to press down with your hands and contract the upper back muscles to open the chest. Walk your feet forward until the legs are straight. Continue to engage your core and glutes to keep your hips lifted. With straight legs, point your toes, reaching the pads of the toes toward the floor.

Chair

Utkatasana

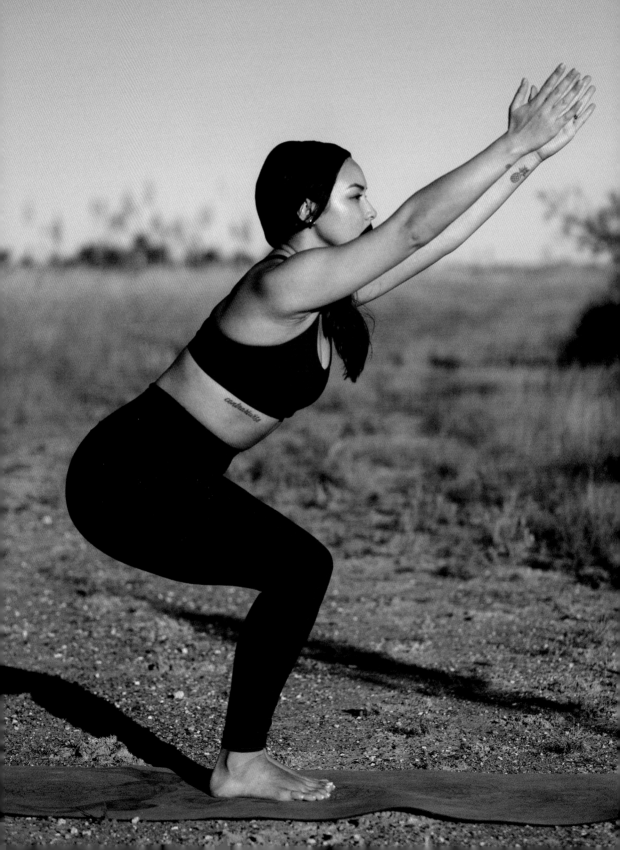

About This Pose

Chair pose is sometimes referred to as fierce pose or awkward chair pose, which seems accurate because it is nowhere near as relaxing as sitting in a chair! It will build strength in your glutes, quadriceps, core, and back extensors. There are different schools of thought as far as keeping a 90-degree angle at your hips or working your thighs parallel to the floor. But more important than the form is the muscular sensation. Find a depth where you feel your glutes activate as you push down through your heels and your entire core is working to keep your spine neutral. If shoulder mobility limits overhead movement, feel free to separate your arms wider, keeping your arms slightly in front or dropping them below shoulder height.

How To

- From mountain pose with feet together or hip-width apart, engage the deep core to stabilize and lift the front of your pelvis.
- Reach your arms overhead and turn the palms to face each other.
- Keeping your toes in contact with the ground, shift your weight back toward your heels and bend your knees to lower your hips to a sitting position. Be sure to align your knees with the midline of your feet: If your feet are together, the knees will be together, and if the feet are hip-width apart, the knees will be over the middle of the feet (don't let your knees touch).
- Push your heels into the ground and activate your glutes as if you were about to stand up.
- Even with the slight natural arch in the lumbar spine, engage your deep core and pull your navel in toward your spine.
- Gaze forward to keep your head in line with the rest of your spine or look up past your hands if that feels comfortable.

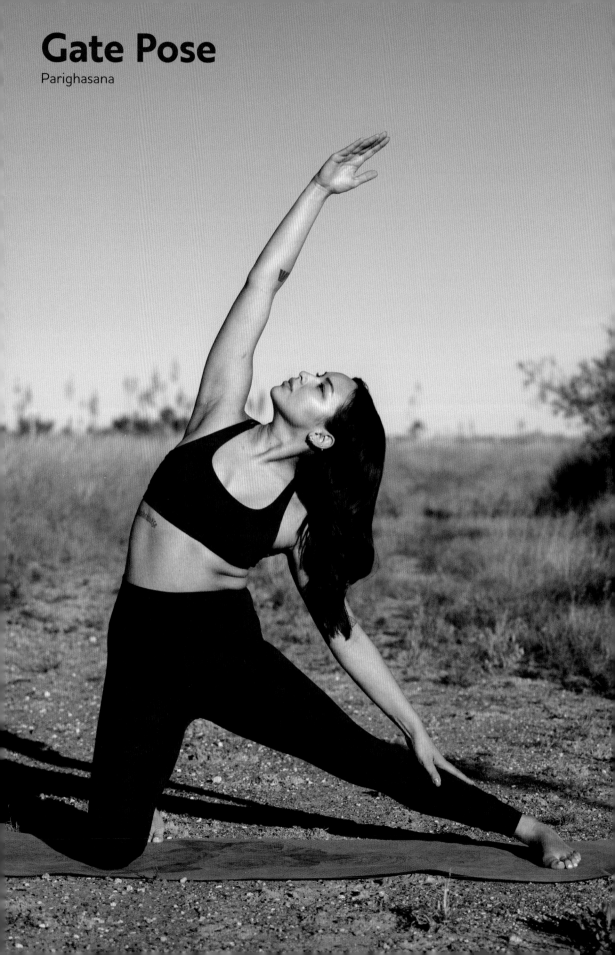

Gate Pose
Parighasana

About This Pose

Gate pose is a lesser sequenced pose that deserves more attention because it has amazing benefits. It stretches both the inner and outer thighs in addition to providing an intense lengthening of the sides of the body. That length prepares you for deep twists, folds, and backbends, as well as opening the side ribs for deeper breathing. Note that in Iyengar yoga, this pose takes both hands to the extended foot. You may eventually work up to that version, but it is not included as a foundational pose. You may want to use a cushion under the knee you are kneeling on.

How To

- From a tall kneeling position, extend one leg out to the side and place your foot completely on the ground, with your toes facing the same direction as your hips.
- Squeeze your glutes and engage your deep core to stabilize your pelvis.
- Slide your same-side arm down your extended leg toward your ankle as far as you can without rotating your chest as you find lateral flexion in the spine.
- Reach your opposite arm overhead with the palm down.
- Inhale and expand the back of your rib cage as well as the top side of your rib cage.
- Exhale and engage the bottom side obliques to access more side bend.
- Gaze forward, keeping your head in line with the rest of your spine, or slightly rotate to look up or down and relax your head.

Crescent Lunge

Ashta Chandrasana

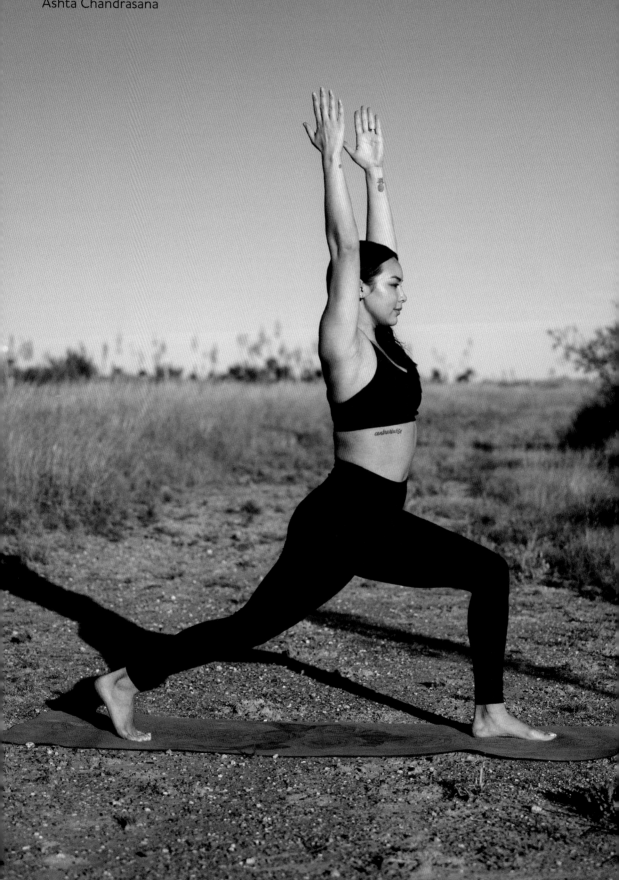

About This Pose

Crescent lunge is a fantastic pose to strengthen your lower body. It stretches the hip flexors of the back leg, which is great if you sit all day or love cycling. The glute of the back leg gains strength in a lengthened position. Crescent lunge will challenge your balance and focus and is a versatile pose to transition into other standing poses.

How To

- From mountain pose, place one foot to the back of your mat into a long lunge, with feet roughly hip-distance apart.
- Adjust the length and depth of your lunge so that your pelvis is neutral and facing forward. Engage the deep core to lift the front of your pelvis and drop your tailbone.
- Stack your front knee over your front heel so you can push down and activate your glute. At the same time, press your back heel into an imaginary wall to engage the glute of your back leg and actively extend your hip.
- Extend your arms overhead, with palms facing each other. Inhale and reach up to lift your rib cage away from your hips.
- Gaze forward or, if it's comfortable on your neck, look up past your hands.

Goddess

Utkata Konasana

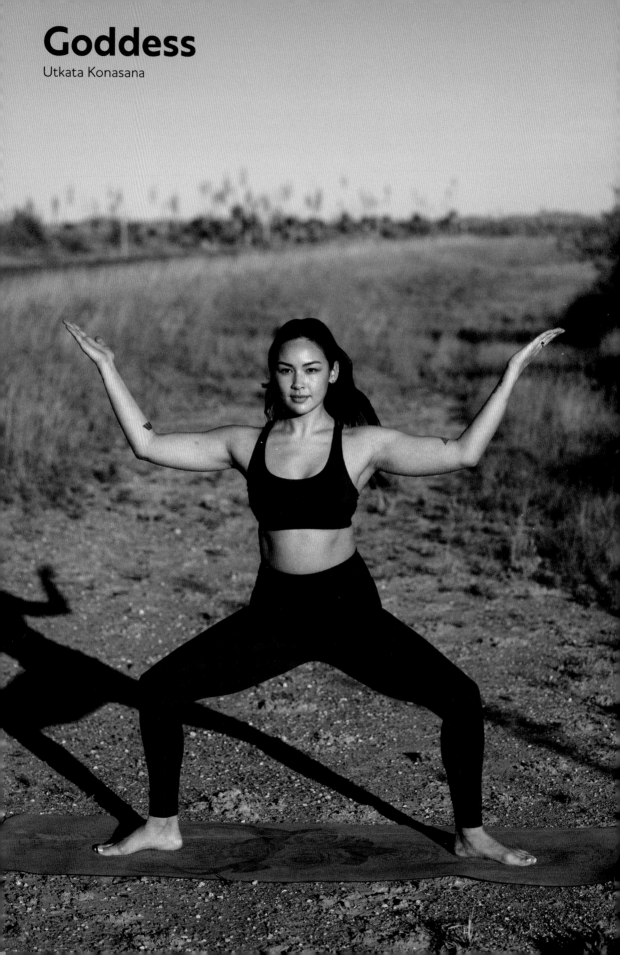

About This Pose

This pose is one with several different names, depending on the school of yoga, and it is sometimes referred to as horse pose, which comes from the fact that your stance is similar to straddling a horse. This standing pose builds strength in your legs, hips, and core while stretching the inner thighs and shoulders.

How To

- Separate your feet wider than your hips and turn your legs out about 45 degrees.
- Keep your spine upright as you bend your knees as if your back is sliding down a wall. Be mindful that your knees follow in the same direction as the toes, and the arches of your feet stay lifted.
- Engage the core and drop your tailbone down to maintain a neutral spine.
- Push your heels into the ground and widen your thighs apart to activate the back and sides of the hips. If you feel only your quadriceps working, check that your knees are not past your toes; you may need to adjust the angles to feel the hips activating.
- Press your palms together at your chest to strengthen your chest and biceps. Alternatively, take your bent arms out to the sides like a cactus or the letter "W" to strengthen your mid back.

Warrior II

Virabhadrasana II

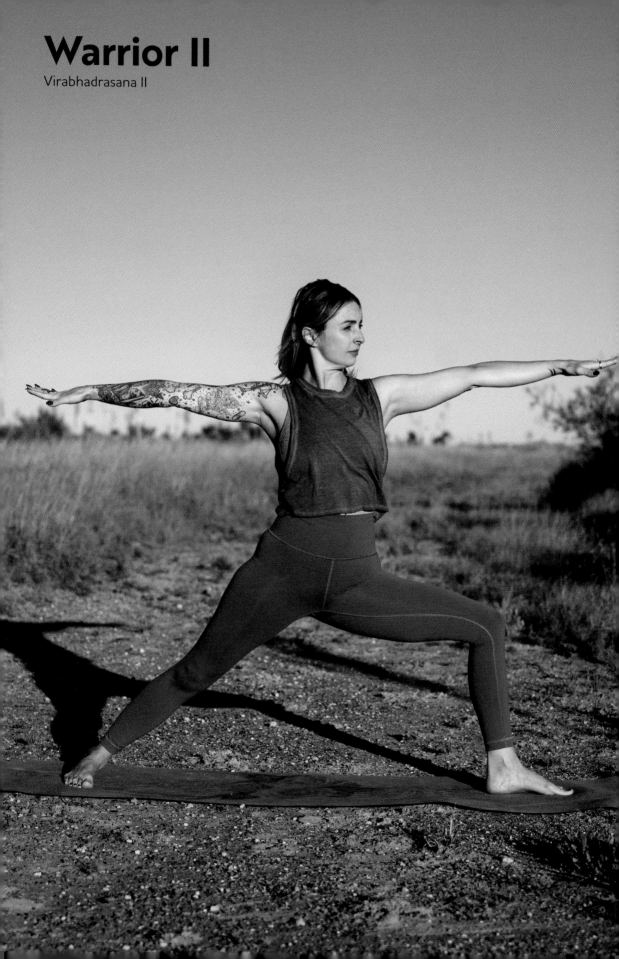

About This Pose

Warrior II is a powerful standing pose that prepares your hips and legs for postures such as side angle and triangle. It strengthens the outer hips, core, and arms while stretching the inner thighs. Here I purposely omitted the common cue of front thigh parallel to the floor because it is more beneficial for the strength and stability of your pelvis for you to focus on maintaining the neutral upright position rather than finding the "correct" depth.

How To

- From crescent lunge, come up about halfway to pivot your back heel down. Allow the hips to turn open to the side as you keep your front foot and knee directed forward and the knee over the heel. The back foot is close to parallel with the back edge of your mat.
- Push down into your heels to activate the glutes as you engage the deep core and lift the pubic bone. This will stabilize your pelvis and can prevent excessive arching in your lower back.
- Turn your chest to face the side of your space and extend your arms out like a "T." Squeeze your triceps and reach out through your fingers.
- Keep your neck long and gaze past your front hand.

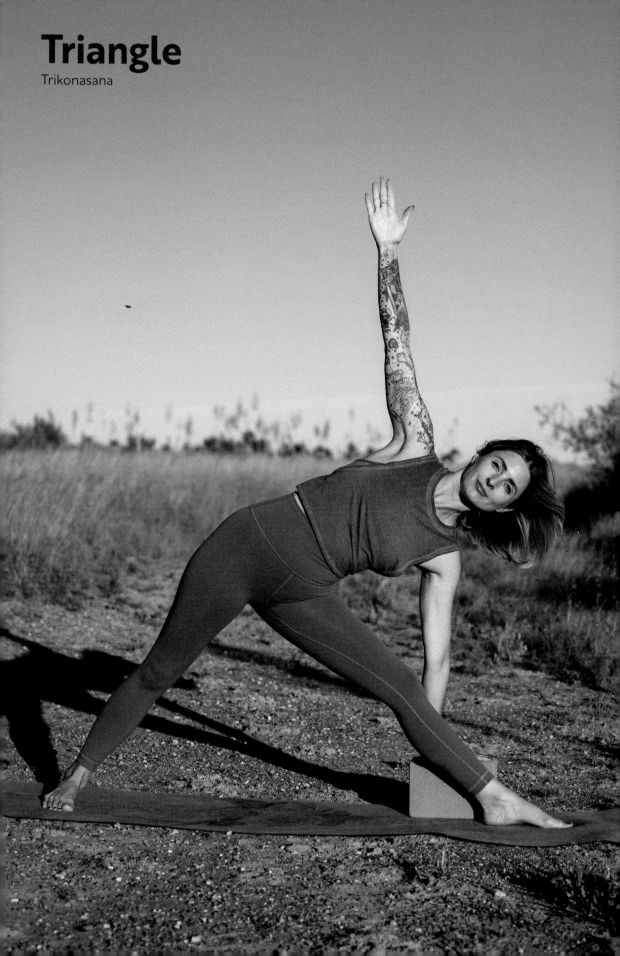

Triangle
Trikonasana

About This Pose

Triangle is a foundational standing pose and stretch for the inner thigh and hamstring of the front leg. It also stretches the outer hip and outer upper thigh of the back leg. The strength of your back leg and oblique muscles work with your supporting arm to hold you up. While many teachers cue front heel in line with the back arch, it is beneficial to align your feet front heel to back heel or even wider, depending on your anatomy.

How To

- From warrior II, engage the quadriceps to straighten your front knee.
- Reach forward with your front arm over the front leg as you pull your front hip back and in toward the inner thigh of your back leg. The hips will now be rotated slightly toward the floor and forward.
- Place your front hand on the floor outside your leg, directly under your shoulder. Use a block if this creates a side body bend or the floor feels too far away. You might also lightly press the back of your hand against the inside of your lower leg. Do not press down on the front of your shin because doing so will likely cause you to lock your knee.
- Extend the top arm straight up, lining up your top hand with your bottom hand, and square your chest to the side of your space.
- Inhale to expand the side ribs and lengthen your spine away from the hips.
- Exhale to engage the deep core. Tighten the muscles of your legs and rotate your bottom rib cage toward the side of your space that you can see.
- Gaze in the same direction as your chest, look down, and relax your neck, or look up past your top hand.

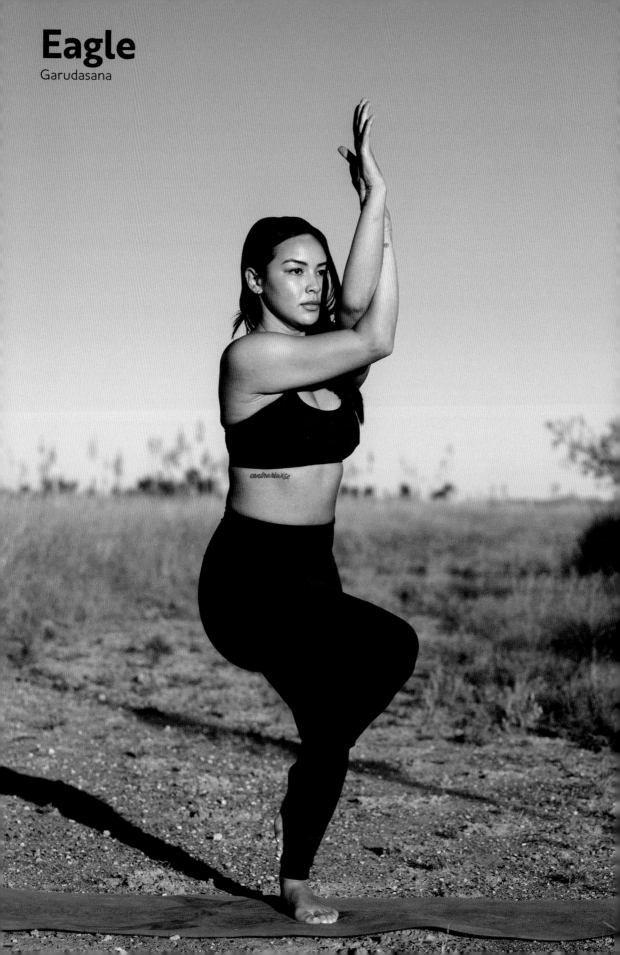

Eagle
Garudasana

About This Pose

Eagle teaches how to balance on one leg while in a compact position, which is generally a more accessible pose. It is also an opportunity to stretch the upper back, trapezius, and outer hips. Eagle strengthens the core, chest, feet, and inner thighs while exploring hip internal rotation—a rare counterpose in the library of standing poses.

How To

- From mountain pose, shift your weight to your left foot as you pull the right knee into your chest. Bend your standing knee and cross your thighs as high up toward your hips as possible. Wrap your floating ankle around the back of your shin.

- Cross your left elbow on top of your right and wrap your forearms so your palms touch, if possible.

- Squeeze your shins against each other side to side and your thighs together top to bottom. Engage the deep core to lift the lower belly. With the bottom knee bent, keep hips low, as in chair pose. Keep the pelvis level across your hip bones.

- Activate the pectoral muscles in your chest by hugging your upper arms tightly to your midline as you press your forearms against one another.

- Inhale deeply to expand your side ribs and between your shoulder blades.

- Gaze forward or at a spot where your forearms touch or close your eyes to challenge your balance.

Downward-Facing Dog

Adho Mukha Svanasana

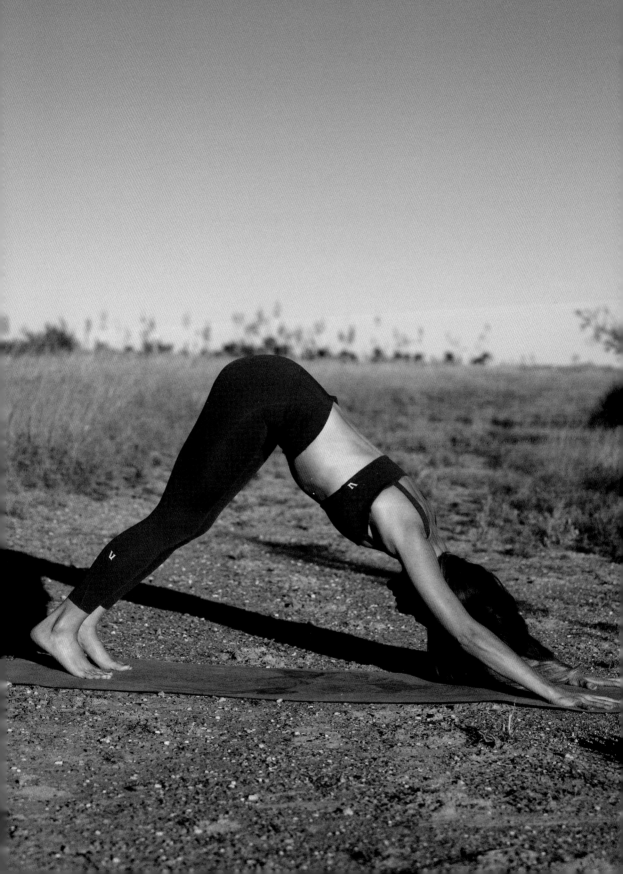

About This Pose

Downward-facing dog, sometimes shortened to down dog, is a full-body pose with many benefits. It stretches the posterior chain—calves, hamstrings, and lats—opens up the chest and shoulders, and introduces inversions, with your heart above your head. It is an integral pose in many styles of yoga, but just because it is repeated frequently does not mean it is easy. Downward-facing dog requires strength in your arms, shoulders, and abdominals to lengthen the spine against the weight of gravity. While the sensations in your upper body will get most of your attention, remember to work your core and legs just as much for the full-body benefits.

How To

- Move into tabletop position, with your hands under your shoulders and your hips a few inches forward of your knees. Spread your fingers wide and grip the ground.
- Tuck your toes, lift your knees, and push your hips up and back so you resemble an upside down "V."
- Push your hands through the floor as you reach your hips back on a diagonal to lengthen the spine.
- Engage your quadriceps and press your thigh bones toward the space behind you. This will create space in front of your hips and hollow out your lower belly.
- Press your heels into or toward the floor to stretch the calves and ankles.
- Inhale into your side ribs and lengthen your spine.
- Exhale from the deep core and relax your head. Gaze between your thighs.
- If your lower back flexes like cat pose, bend your knees, point your heels high, or adjust the length of your dog until you find a version where you have a natural curve in your spine.

Dolphin
Ardha Pincha Mayurasana

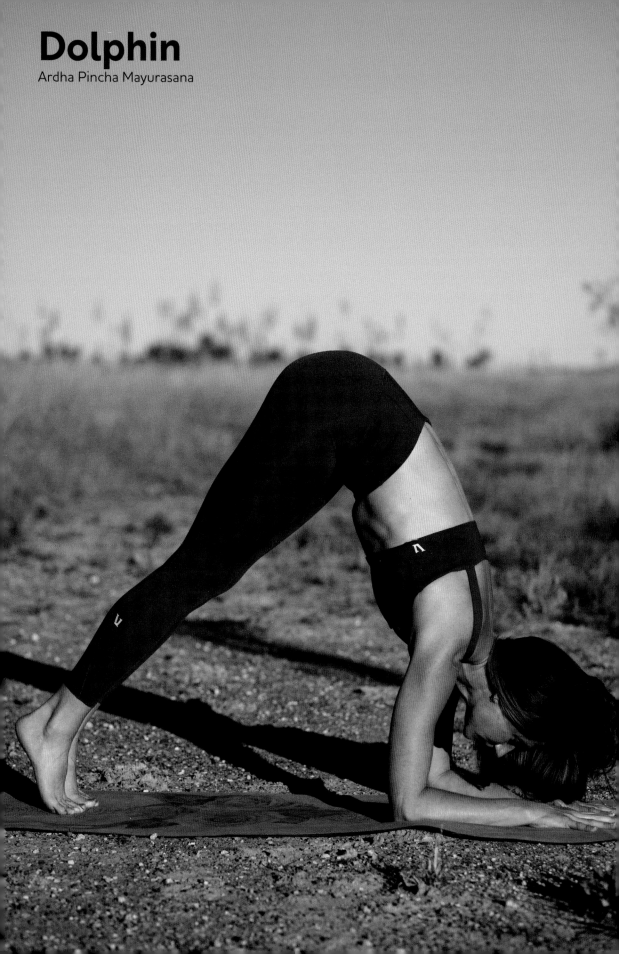

About This Pose

Dolphin is essentially downward-facing dog on your forearms. This is a wonderful option if your wrists need a rest; however, it is much less forgiving on shoulder mobility, so most people find it feels more challenging. Like downward-facing dog, this pose builds strength primarily in the shoulders with the added intensity of deeper core connection and activation while stretching the hamstrings, calves, and latissimus muscles. You also get the benefits of an inversion—improved circulation and energy, among others—without bearing weight on your head.

How To

- From tabletop position, place your elbows on the floor underneath your shoulders. If your shoulder mobility allows, separate your forearms parallel and place your palms flat. Otherwise, interlace your fingers and press the pinky edges of your hands into the ground.

- Gaze between your forearms as if you are preparing for full forearm stand, or relax your head down. Push your elbows and wrists firmly into the floor and squeeze your elbows toward each other.

- Point your heels high and bend your knees slightly to allow room to walk your feet closer to your hands. Eventually, your hips will stack over your shoulders and elbows. However, you want to maintain as much length in the spine and as little rounding in the lower back as possible.

- Engage the deep core to lift your hips up and bring the bottom ribs up to maintain a neutral spine. This rib cage position may feel more challenging for your shoulder strength, especially if you are quite flexible—but resist the temptation to move your chest into a backbend.

- Continuously push down through your shoulders and breathe deeply to expand the side ribs and back ribs.

Hero

Virasana

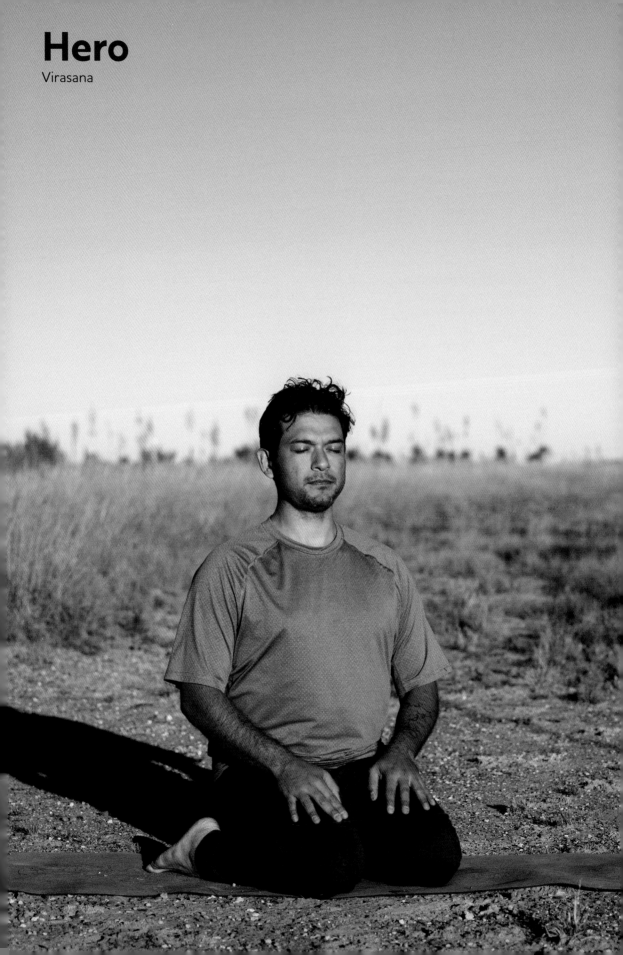

About This Pose

Hero is a variation on vajrasana, or thunderbolt, pose. However, rather than sitting on your heels, separate the feet and sit between your heels. This small change makes a big difference because it requires more internal rotation at the hip and the knee joints. Hero stretches the front of the ankles and quadriceps, and the reclined variation (found in the Restorative Poses section), supta virasana, adds a deep psoas stretch to make it a fairly advanced pose. Hero is a fantastic stretch for the quadriceps if you love cycling or running, and many yogis find it more accessible than comfortable pose (sukhasana) to sit tall without collapsing the lower back.

How To

- In a tall kneeling position with the knees together, separate your feet slightly wider than hip-distance apart.
- Place your hips on the floor between your feet. Tilt your pelvis slightly forward and back until you find the midpoint where your pelvis is neutral and your lumbar spine can move into its natural curve.
- Keep the bottom ribs down as you bring the shoulder blades softly back and down and open the collarbones. Lengthen the entire spine from tailbone to crown to create as much length in your torso as possible in this seated position.
- Gaze at the floor in front of you or close your eyes for meditation.

Variation

Hero Pose With Bolster

Follow the instructions of hero pose, but instead of sitting directly on the floor, place the short edge of a bolster under your hips. Your shins and feet will be along the outside of the bolster, with your toes pointing behind you.

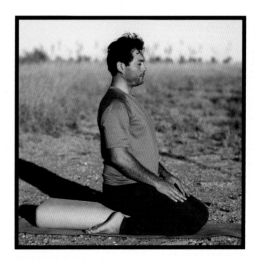

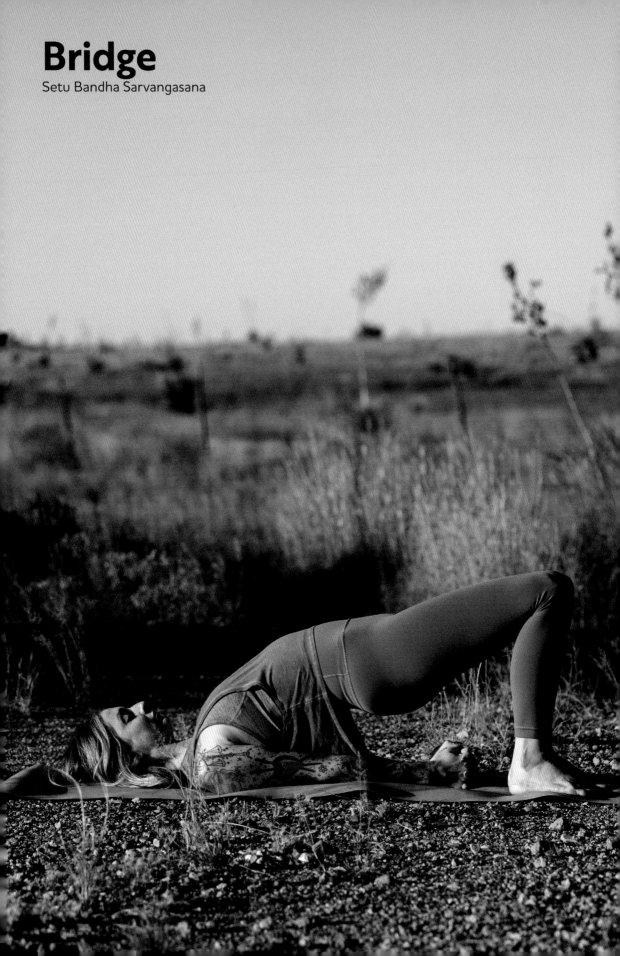

Bridge
Setu Bandha Sarvangasana

About This Pose

Bridge is a reclined backbend using your legs and arms pushing into the ground to lift yourself up. It stretches the quadriceps, hip flexors, abdominals, and chest while preparing you for deeper backbends such as upward-facing bow. Bridge builds strength in the hamstrings, glutes, and back extensors—including the erector spinae and latissimus. Everything in the back of your body is contracting to stretch everything in the front.

How To

- Lie down on your back with the knees bent and place your feet roughly hip-distance apart—close enough to your hips that you can touch your heels with your fingertips. When you lift up, your heels will be directly under your knees.

- Push your feet down and squeeze your glutes to lift the hips. Engage the lower core and bring the pubic bone toward your navel while reaching your tailbone toward the backs of your knees once your hips are lifted off the floor.

- With your arms long by your sides, push your arms and shoulders into the ground to lift your chest toward your chin. Gaze straight up and avoid looking left or right.

- Position your shoulders more underneath you until you can interlace your fingers and press your wrists strongly into the floor.

- Push the back of your head down as you keep a slight tuck of your chin.

- Inhale to expand the rib cage and pull your chest closer to your chin.

- Exhale and contract the hamstrings, glutes, and muscles in your mid and upper back to deepen the backbend.

- Lengthen your chest and knees in opposite directions to stretch the front of your body as you lift your hips up.

Yogi Squat
Malasana

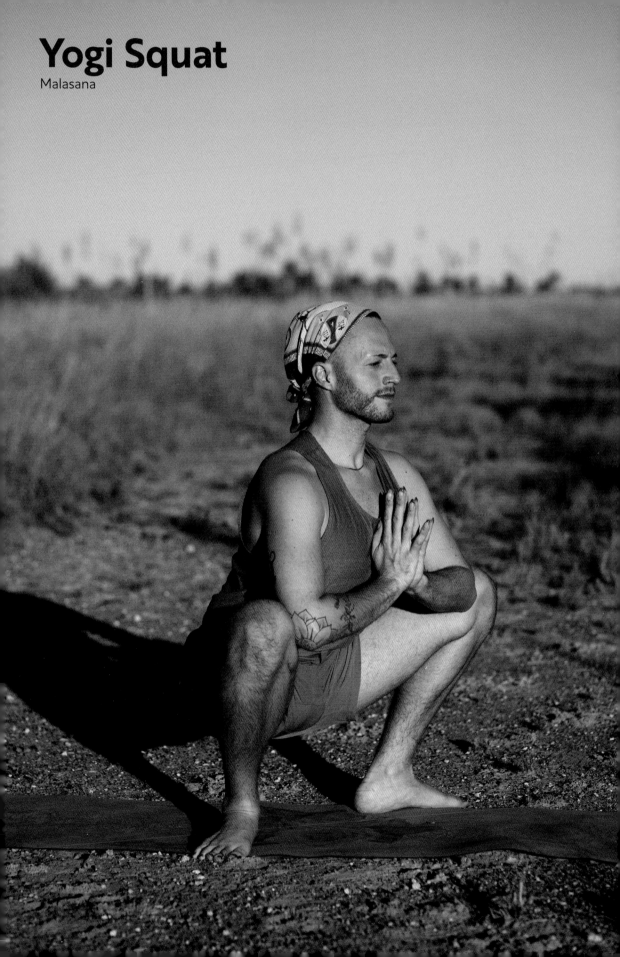

About This Pose

Also known as garland, this is a deep stretch for the inner hips, legs, and feet. It builds strength in the front of the shins and ankles, outer hips, and core. Functionally, this pose can assist in relaxing the pelvic floor, and it aids the digestive process. Hip structure varies widely, so adjust the angles of your legs and depth of your hips as needed. Spend time building endurance and ease with this version, and then feel free to try variations such as a support squat (see variation photo) or flexed spine.

How To

- Standing in mountain pose, separate your feet wider than your hips and perhaps angle your feet slightly outward. Bend your knees and lower your hips into a squat with heels on the ground.
- As you sink your hips low, shift more weight onto your heels and reach the crown of your head straight up to lengthen the spine and to prevent rounding in your back. Drop your shoulders away from your ears. For a counterbalance to avoid falling backward, you may reach your arms forward.
- Place your palms together at your chest and gently rest your elbows against your inner thighs. Resist the urge to widen your thighs. For several breaths, squeeze your legs into your arms and engage the deep core. On an exhale, relax and gently open your knees to deepen the stretch on your inner legs.

Variation

Supported Yogi Squat

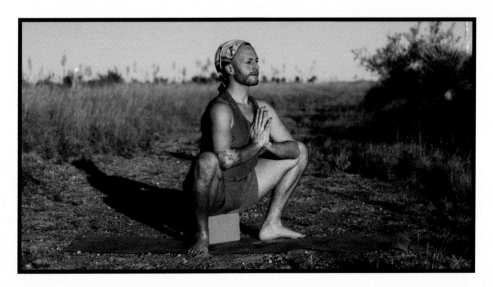

If your balance feels compromised in the yogi squat or to take pressure off the knees and hips, place a block or two under the sitz bones to support your body weight. Continue to aim the crown of your head up toward the sky in an attempt to lengthen your spine. Engage your core to find an upward lift in the chest. Keep the shoulders relaxed and the palms together at the center of the chest. Engage your outer thighs to bring the knees wide of center.

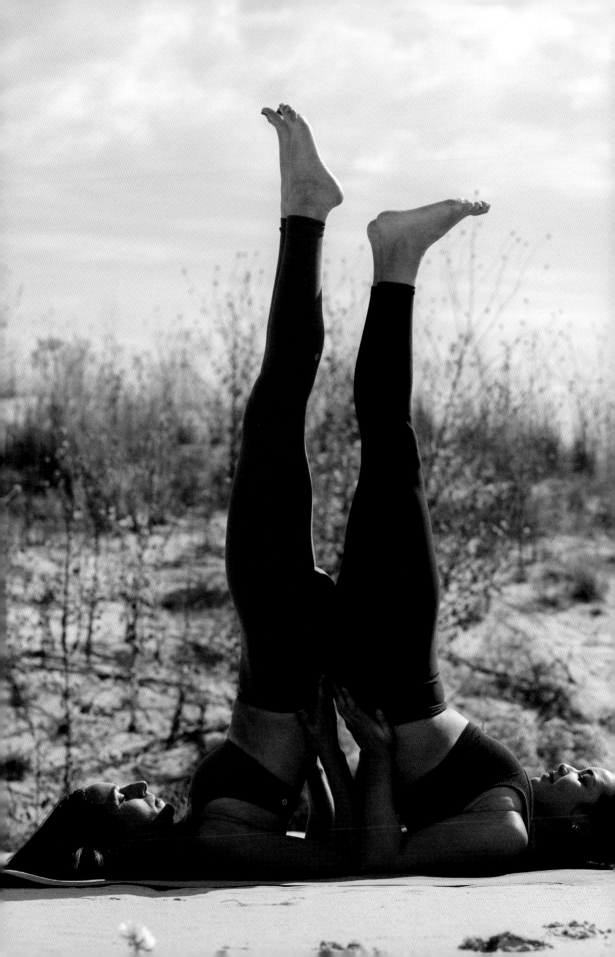

PART II
DEEPEN

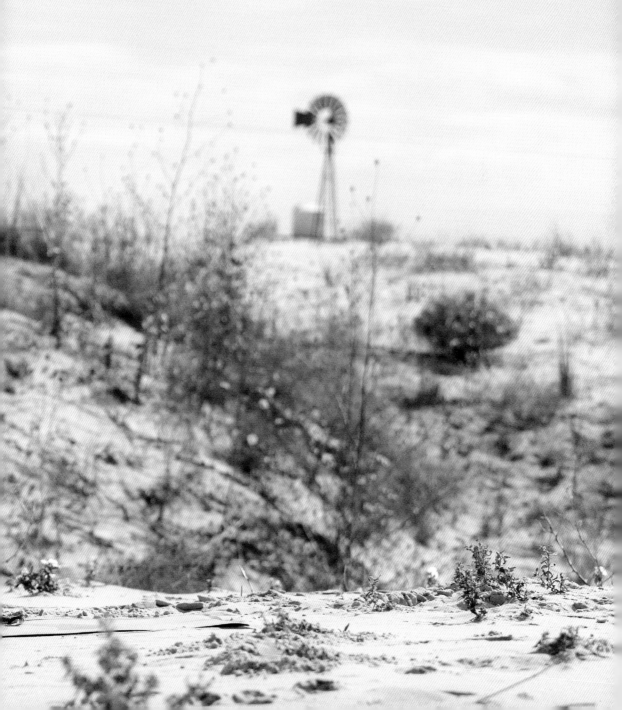

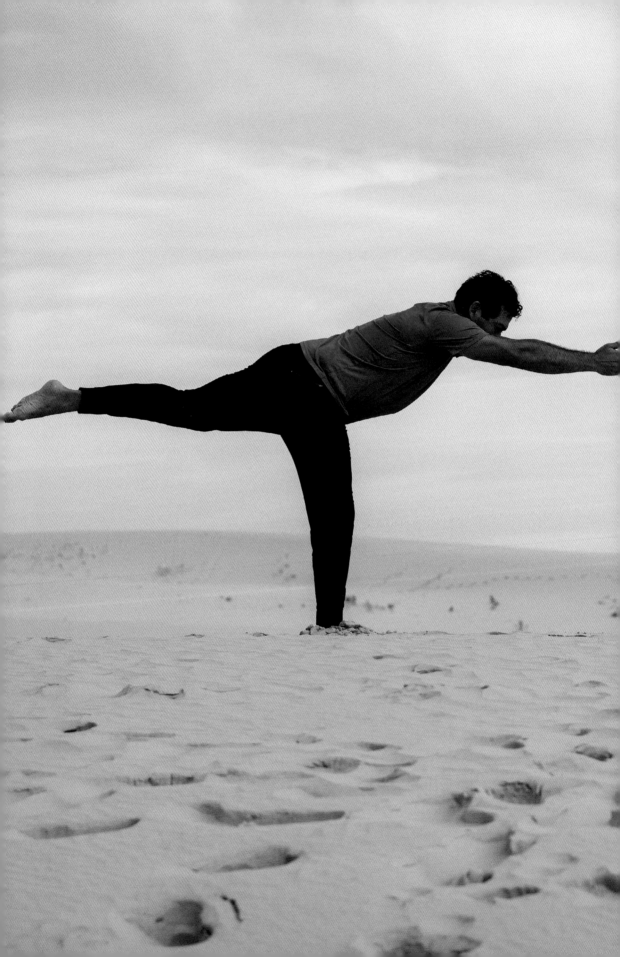

3

STANDING POSES

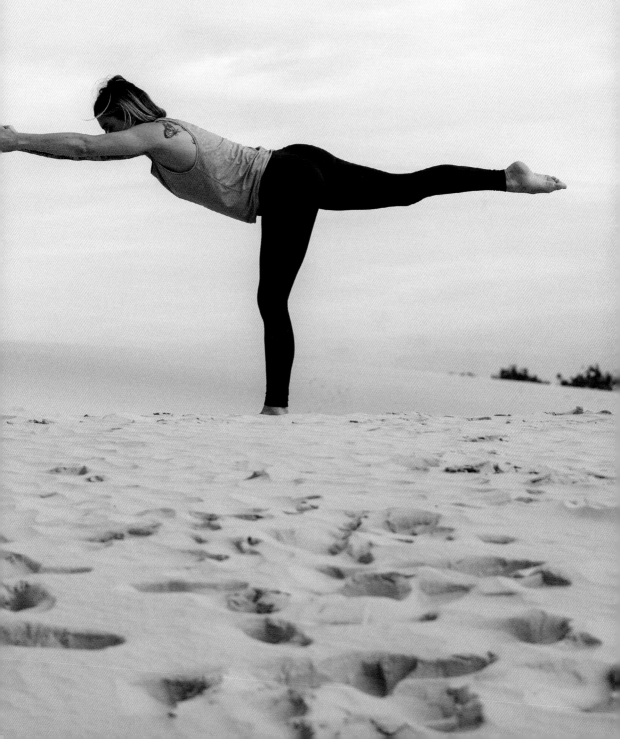

Warrior I
Virabhadrasana I

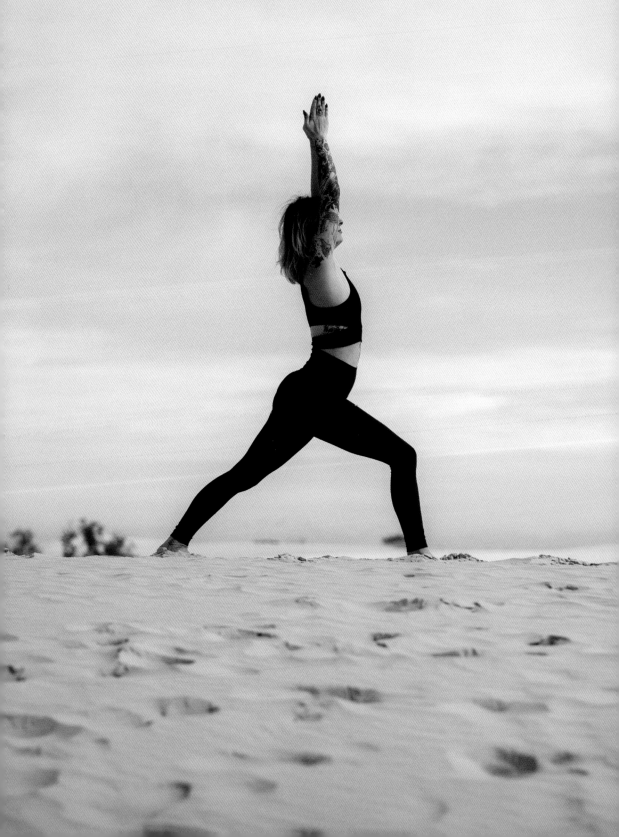

About This Pose

While many consider this a level 1 or foundational pose, it is a challenging one, with several opposing actions that require great strength and mobility to execute well. Warrior I strengthens and stretches both legs in opposite ways—lengthening the front of the back leg and strengthening the back of the front leg. Deep core strength is necessary to maintain stability and balance while keeping the spine lifted. Shoulder mobility is also required to reach the arms overhead.

How To

- From mountain pose, step one foot back into a lunge, with your feet roughly hip-distance apart. A wider stance will feel more stable.
- Pivot your heel to the ground and angle your toes toward the front corner of your mat at whatever degree is comfortable for your ankle and knee.
- Bend your front knee and push both heels into the ground to activate the glutes.
- Engage your deep core and attempt to drop your tailbone toward the floor. In this separated leg stance, the movement will be subtle but powerful.
- Inhale and lift your entire rib cage away from your hips while extending your arms overhead.
- If it is possible with straight arms and no pain, press your palms together overhead and look up to your thumbs. Another option is arms parallel or even wider into a small "V" shape.
- From your glutes to your feet, push down as you reach your upper body upward.

Humble Warrior

Baddha Virabhadrasana

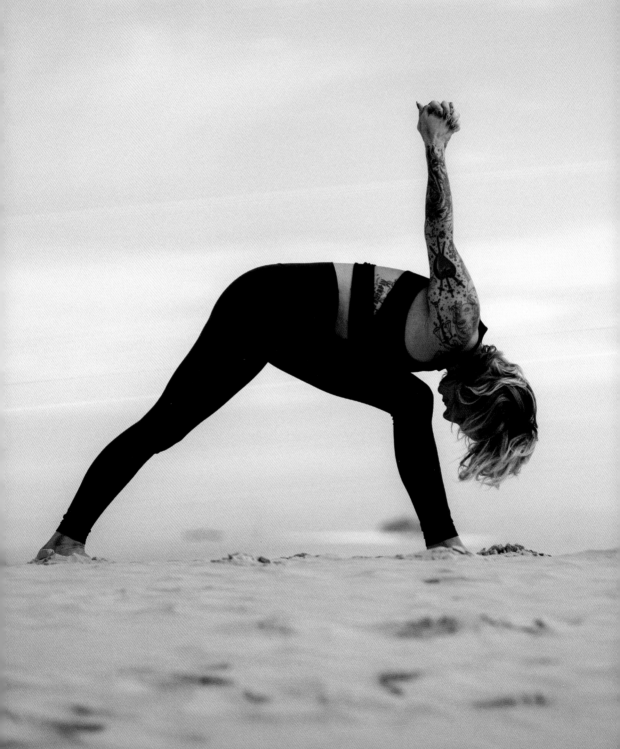

About This Pose

This more recent variation on warrior I requires just as much strength as the upright pose but in different ways. As you bow into the flexibility of the hips and legs, you must access the inner thighs and deep core to resist collapsing the torso toward the floor when you are folded forward. The shoulder extension arm bind stretches the pectorals and biceps.

How To

- From warrior I pose, separate your feet slightly wider than hip distance to create more space to flex at the hip.
- Interlace your fingers behind your lower back. Depending on your anatomy and mobility, you can press the palms together or allow them to separate, but your grip should remain firm and triceps engaged.
- Inhale and lengthen the rib cage away from your hips as you press down into your feet.
- Keep your legs engaged, with the back heel still pressing down into the floor, fold forward toward the inside of your front leg, and drop your head toward the floor, flexing the spine.
- Lift up on the pelvic floor and lower core so there is a sense of drawing energy in and up rather than sinking down.
- Squeeze the upper back muscles between your shoulder blades. Reach out through your knuckles and lift your hands away from your hips.

Side Angle
Parsvakonasana

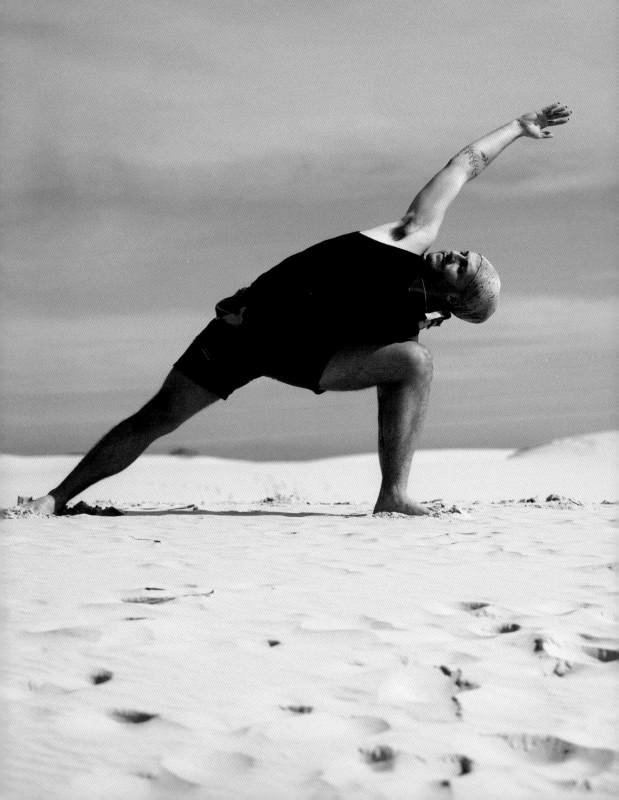

About This Pose

We can view this pose as a variation on warrior II (changing the upper-body angle) or a variation on triangle (changing the front knee angle). Either way, this pose requires strength in both legs and the core while providing a deep stretch for the entire top side of the body and the back of the front leg.

How To

- From warrior II, keep the chest squared off to the side of your space as you hinge your torso over your front leg.
- Place your bottom hand outside your front foot. Squeeze your arm and leg against each other to activate the outer hip muscles as you push down through your back foot.
- Press the outer edge of your back foot into the floor and reach your top arm overhead with your bicep above your top ear, creating a diagonal line from your foot to your hand.
- Even as you press down into both feet, isometrically drag your feet toward each other to strengthen the inner thighs and create stability in the hip joints.
- Allow your gaze to follow the direction of your sternum, or if it is comfortable on your neck, look up from underneath your top arm.

Variation

Side Angle With Extended Arms

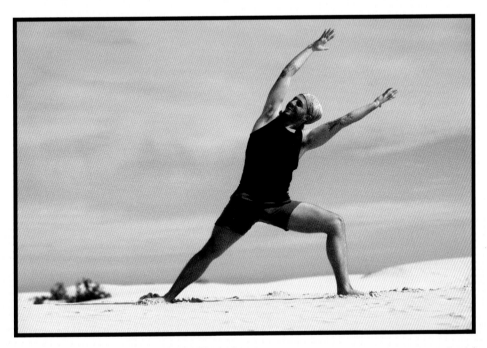

Reach both arms alongside your head, with the biceps framing the ears to build greater strength in your legs and core.

Revolved Side Angle

Parivrtta Parsvakonasana

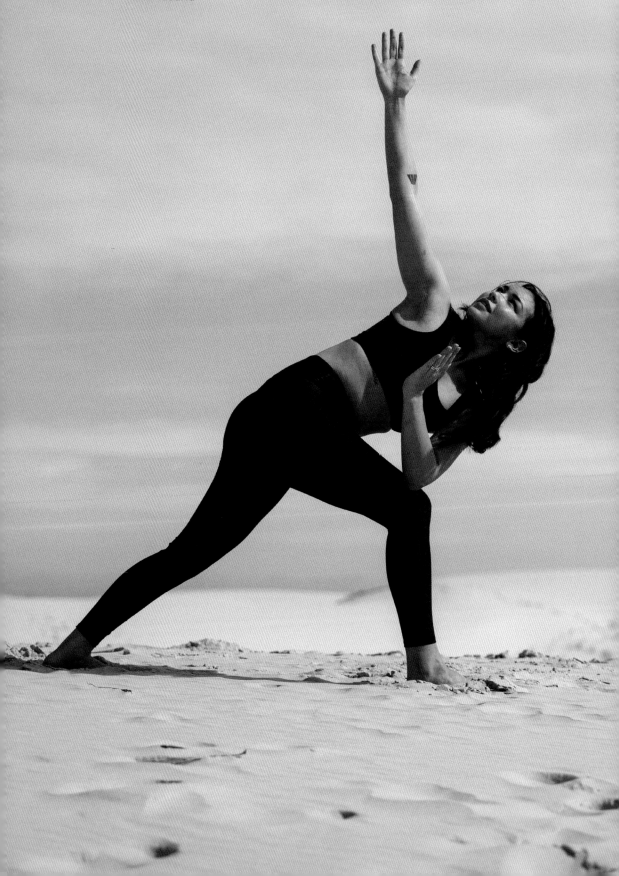

About This Pose

Although the pose name is revolved side angle, the pelvis position is more akin to warrior I. The back heel on the ground intensifies the sensation of the spinal twist, yet it can be more stable for the pelvis because you can press down more using the strength of your lower body.

How To

- From warrior I on the right side, place your right hand on your right thigh to anchor your hip. Reach your left arm up and across on a diagonal to maximize the length in the left side for the twist.
- As you rotate your rib cage over your front thigh, hook your left arm on the outside of your right thigh and either keep your bottom elbow bent (pictured) or place your left hand on the ground next to your front foot.
- Press the back of your upper left arm against the outside of your front thigh and simultaneously press your thigh against your arm.
- Externally rotate your right arm as you reach that arm overhead.
- As you inhale, lengthen the rib cage away from the hips.
- As you exhale, press down into your feet with strong legs and twist more through the rib cage. The resistance of your thigh and your arm will create additional leverage into the twist, and it also creates stability in the front hip.
- Allow your gaze to follow the direction of your sternum, or if it is comfortable on your neck, look up from underneath your top arm.

Variation

Revolved Lunge

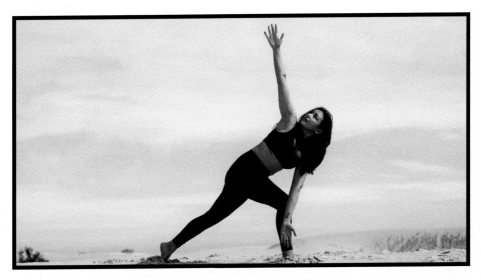

If you are having trouble keeping your back heel on the ground, follow the instructions for revolved side angle but lift your back heel in alignment over the ball of the foot. The toes of the back foot will now point forward instead of out at 45 degrees, as in revolved side angle. This variation will also allow your hips to be squarer with the front of the mat, taking pressure off the back knee and lower back.

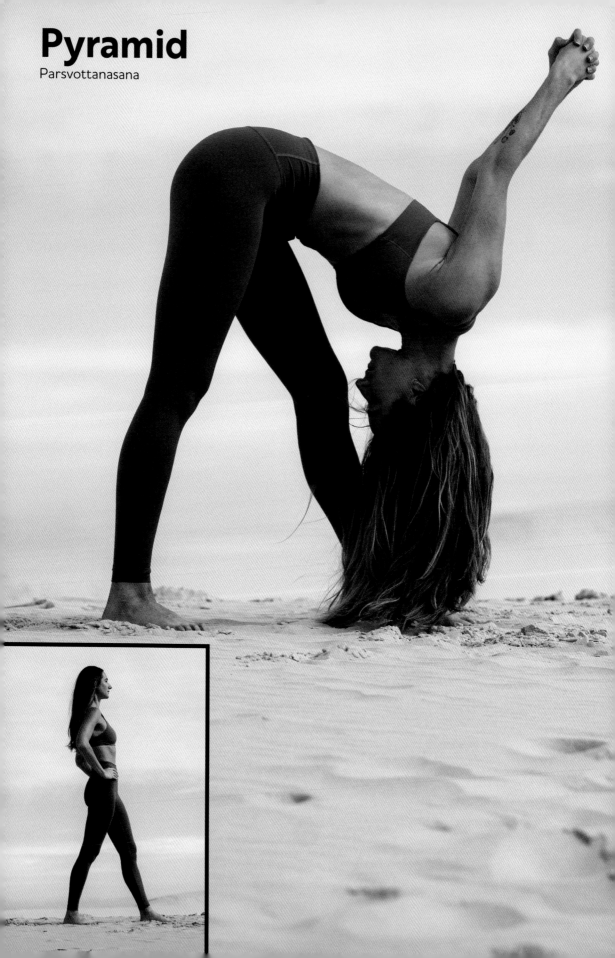

Pyramid
Parsvottanasana

About This Pose

Pyramid pose always ranks as one of my top poses for any yoga asana practice. It builds strength in your legs and core while stretching the posterior chain. Stability in the lower body allows you to lengthen and stretch the spine, especially the lumbar. Although this neutral spine variation is more common (and, for a new student, I would introduce this one first), a rounded spine version with the forehead to the knee is beneficial for stretching the entirety of the back line of the body and fascia. It also requires intense deep core engagement but could be contraindicated for some back issues.

How To

- From mountain pose, place your hands on your hips for tactile feedback to keep your hips squared forward.
- Step one foot back one-third to one-half the length of your mat. Line up your feet so they are roughly hip-distance apart, with the back foot angled toward the front corner of your mat (at a 45-degree angle) of the same side as the back foot.
- Engage your quadriceps to lift the kneecaps and push down into the ground with both feet.
- Inhale and lengthen the rib cage away from your hips as you reach your arms out to the sides like a "T."
- Exhale and internally rotate your biceps so they face down and back. Bend your elbows and clasp your wrists behind your back or press the palms together in reverse prayer.
- Keep lengthening the spine away from your hips as you hinge forward.
- Engage your core muscles and pull your low abdomen inward toward your spine, and imagine squeezing your legs together as you press down into the ground.
- Inhale to expand the back and side ribs as you lengthen the spine.
- Gaze at your front foot or shin.

Variation

Pyramid With Blocks

If you are having trouble with your balance with your hands behind your back, place a yoga block under each hand as high as you need to be able to press down into the blocks while lengthening both legs by engaging your quadriceps.

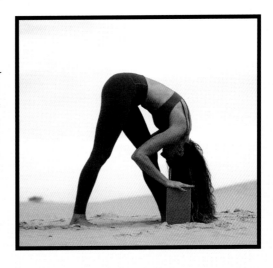

Revolved Triangle
Parivrtta Trikonasana

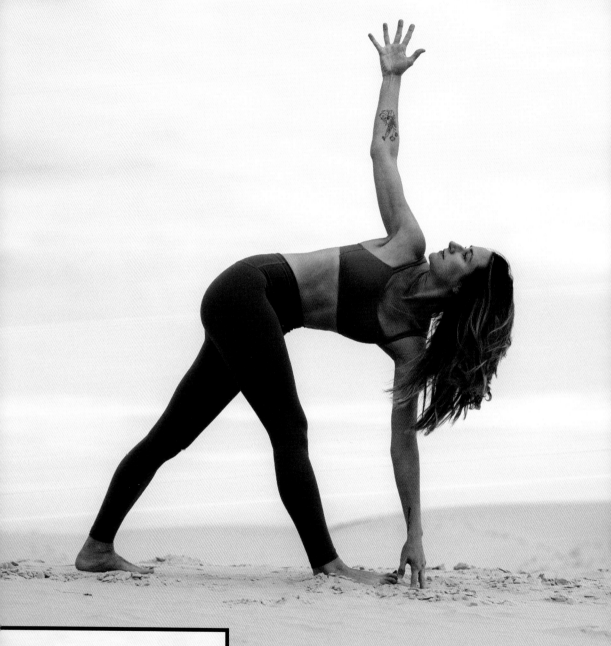

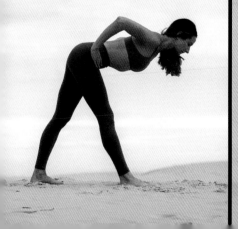

About This Pose

Although the name of this pose implies a variation on triangle, the lower body and pelvis position is more akin to that of pyramid pose. This challenging spinal twist pose builds strength in the legs and core while stretching the hamstrings, lateral hips, and chest.

How To

- From mountain pose with your feet hip-width apart, place your hands on your hips. With your left foot, step approximately halfway back on your mat and pivot your heel to the ground, toes pointing out 45 degrees toward the front corner of the mat on the same side as your back foot. Your heels will be roughly hip-distance apart rather than like walking a tightrope.
- Use the quadriceps to lift your kneecaps and engage the lower core to stabilize your pelvis.
- As you inhale, elevate the ribs away from your hips.
- As you exhale, fold forward over your front leg, with the core engaged.
- Place your left hand on the ground next to the pinky-toe side of your front (right) foot.
- Simultaneously push down into your feet and squeeze the inner thighs in and up.
- Push your hand into the ground and stretch your right arm upward. Exhale as you turn the back left rib cage toward the right side of your space.
- Gaze past your top hand.

Half Moon
Ardha Chandrasana

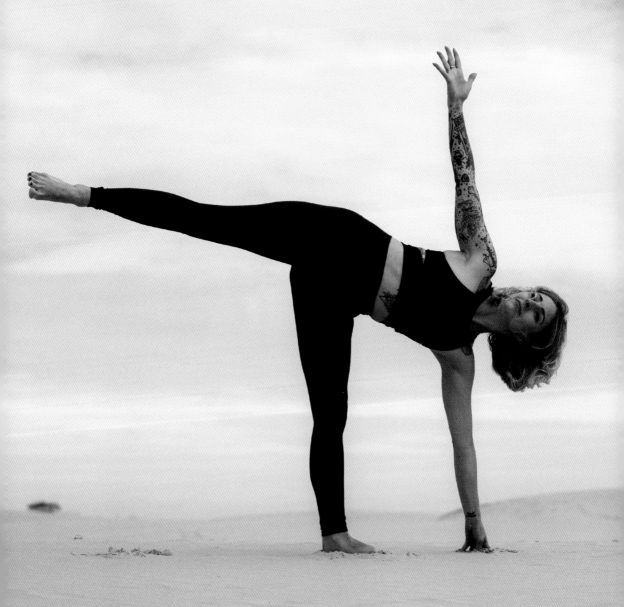

About This Pose

Half moon is essentially triangle with the added challenge of balancing on one leg. For that reason, it builds strength in the outer hip of the standing leg and stability through the core muscles, especially the obliques.

How To

- From warrior II, shift your weight more forward onto your front leg.
- Reach your hand on the same side as your front leg down to the floor in front of your foot and push into your front heel to lift the back leg up to hip height.
- Although your hips will not be *exactly* parallel to the side of your space, do stack the top hip bone above the bottom hip bone by engaging the outer hip muscles of your standing leg and pushing firmly through the heel.
- Make your elevated leg straight and strong while using the gluteus medius on the side of your hip to lift the leg and foot in line with you hip socket.
- Stretch up through the top arm to lift and rotate your chest.
- Squeeze the muscles in your arms and legs to keep them strong and expand out in all directions.
- Gaze down at the ground in the same direction as your chest or up past your top hand.

Variation

Candy Cane

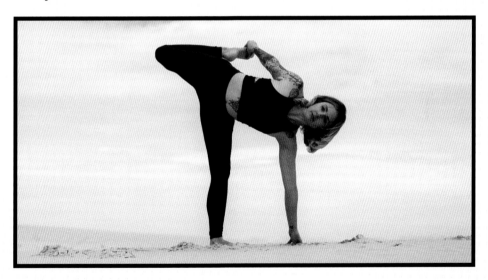

From half moon, bend the knee of the elevated leg, engaging your hamstring, as if you are doing a hamstring curl, to pull your foot toward your glute. Grab hold of your top foot with your top hand and press your foot back into your hand and away from your glute to stretch the hip flexor and quadricep. Keep the top outer knee in line with the top outer hip instead of letting the knee lift upward.

Revolved Half Moon

Parivrtta Ardha Chandrasana

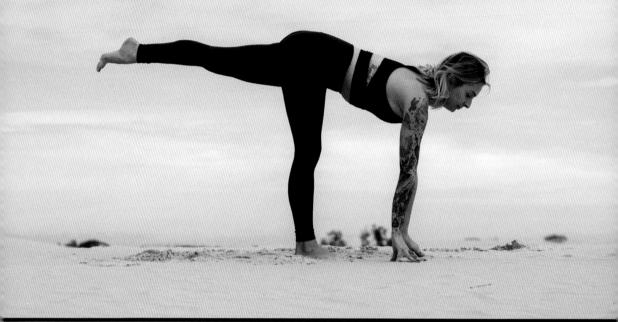

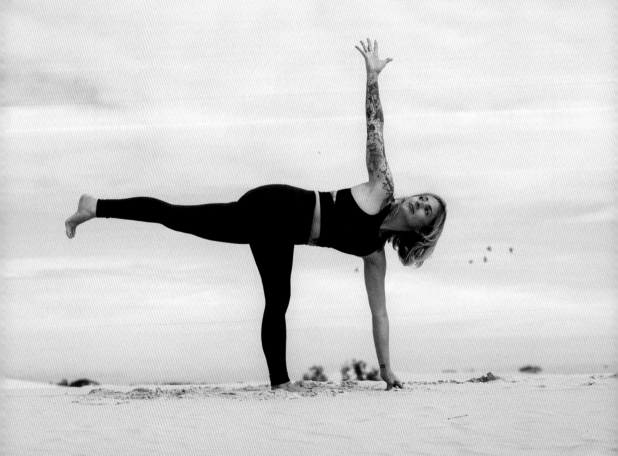

About This Pose

In many ways, revolved half moon pose is a variation on revolved triangle pose. It requires similar actions and strength in the legs, hips, and core—all while balancing on one foot.

How To

- From pyramid pose on the right side, shift your weight more forward into your front (right) leg and squeeze the glute to lift your back (left) leg like with warrior III (see next pose).
- Walk your hands forward until your hips are over your standing leg and your hands are under your shoulders.
- Engage the quadriceps to lift the kneecaps and isometrically press your standing foot out to the right to activate the muscles that stabilize the outer hip.
- Engage the deep core and squeeze the glutes to stabilize the pelvis and create the strength to balance.
- Keep the left hand grounded as you reach your right hand upward and turn from your back left rib cage.
- Push down into the ground with your hand as you stretch up and out through the top arm. This may allow you to twist deeper.
- Turn your gaze to follow the direction of your chest, or if it is comfortable on your neck, look up past your top hand.

Warrior III
Virabhadrasana III

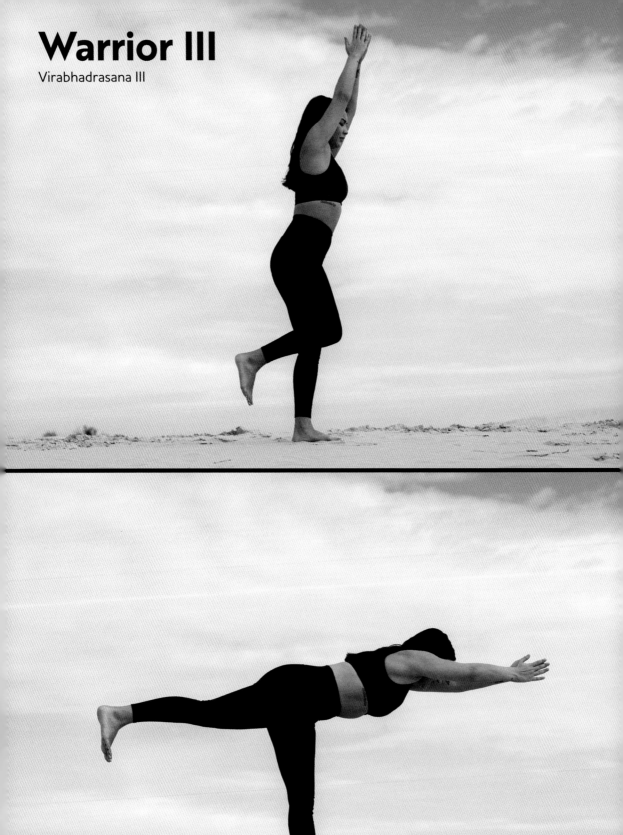

About This Pose

While warrior III may look like a straightforward pose, it is deceptively tricky. The long lever of your arms overhead combined with balancing on one leg requires both a contracting in (by engaging your core) and an expanding out (by stretching through your arms and legs in opposite directions).

How To

- From mountain pose, extend the arms overhead, strong and straight. Press the palms together if your shoulder mobility allows; otherwise, your hands can be shoulder-distance apart.
- Shift your weight to one foot and softly bend that knee. This will wake up the muscles in your leg and assist with balance.
- Press down into your heel while the toes remain in contact with the floor.
- Hinge forward at the hips and extend your elevated leg behind you until you create a "T" shape with your entire body, keeping the arms extended overhead.
- Engage the deep core to keep your torso lifting up away from the ground, and squeeze your glutes.
- Like you were the rope in a game of "tug of war," stretch your hands and your elevated leg in opposite directions.
- Focus your gaze on a point on the ground below.

Variation

Airplane

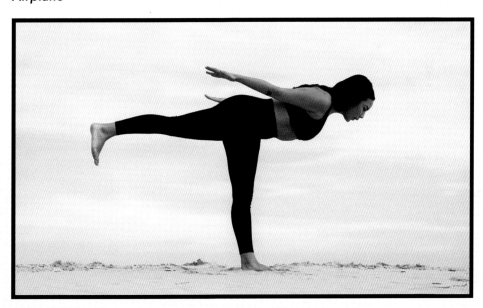

Sweep your arms by your hips and squeeze your shoulder blades together. To keep the core tight, resist the urge to do a backbend.

Forward Fold
Uttanasana

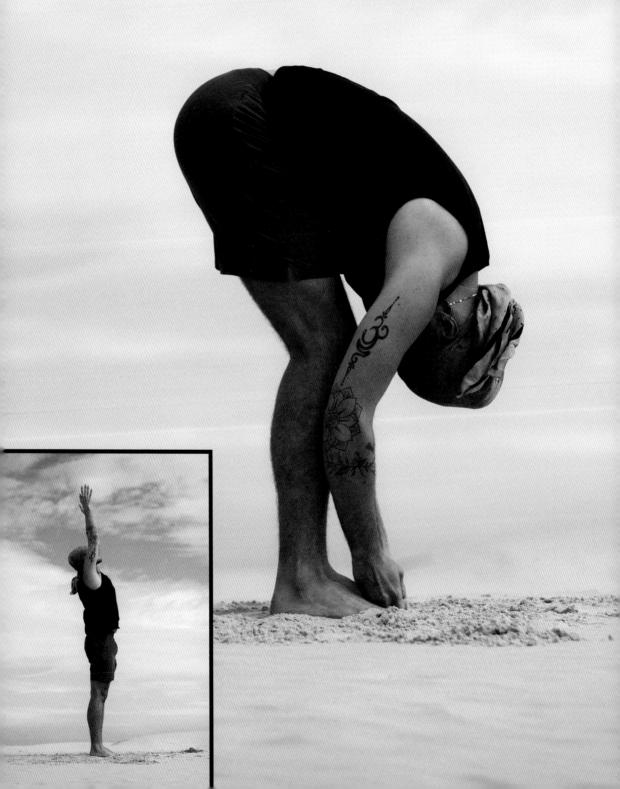

About This Pose

Forward fold uses the strength of the front of the body to stretch the posterior chain. Although gravity and your arms offer some assistance, major strength can be built in the quadriceps, hip flexors, and core by actively contracting to deepen the forward fold. Half-lift forward fold (ardha uttanasana) is part of the sun salutation sequence and teaches you to keep a straight spine and bend exclusively from the hips (see variation photos).

How To

- From mountain pose, with feet hip-width apart or wider, inhale and stretch your arms overhead.
- Exhale to engage the lower core and hinge forward at your hips.
- Grab your big toes with the first two fingers of each hand or place your hands on the ground next to your feet outside the pinky toes.
- Inhale to expand the back and sides of your rib cage.
- As you exhale, hollow out the lower belly as if you are trying to fit a soccer ball between your abdomen and thighs.
- At the same time, with or without the assistance of your hands, engage the hip flexors to bring your upper body closer to your legs.
- Reach the crown of your head toward the space between your feet on the floor.

Variations

Half-Lift Forward Fold

From forward fold, if the hamstrings allow, place your fingertips in line outside the edges of your toes. Without locking your knees, engage the quadriceps. As you inhale, lengthen the spine, moving the crown of the head forward with your gaze on the ground. Engage the core, lifting your navel toward your spine to support and lengthen the back. Bring your shoulders back from the ears and pull your shoulder blades in toward the spine to keep your chest broad and open.

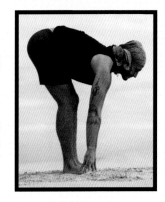

Half-Lift Forward Fold With Hands to Shins

If keeping your fingers on the floor outside of the toes prevents you from straightening your legs, you may modify this pose, with your hands lightly pressing onto your shins (do not push into your shins—just place your hands on your shins, below your knees). Inhale while lifting halfway up to align your back parallel to the sky. Bring your shoulder blades softly back and down to broaden the collarbone and extend your neck. Keep your core engaged, lifting your navel to your spine, and find axial extension from your tailbone to your crown as if you are lengthening your spine both forward and back at the same time. Keep the quadriceps engaged without locking the knees.

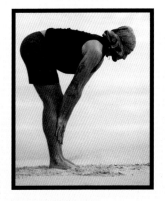

Standing Hand to Big Toe

Utthita Hasta Padangusthasana

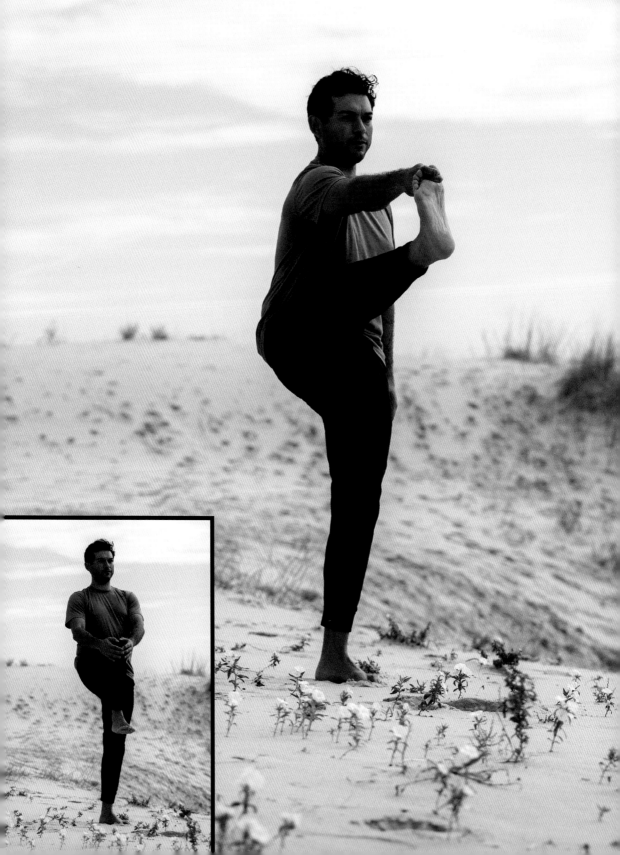

About This Pose

Also known as standing extended-leg stretch, this balancing pose requires opposing actions in the legs—using the strength in the back of the standing hip and leg while stretching the back of the lifted leg.

How To

- From mountain pose, shift your weight to one foot and softly bend that knee to engage the muscles of the leg and assist with balance.
- Set your gaze on something stationary in front of you.
- Use the deep core to stabilize your pelvis as you move your opposite knee into your chest. Hold your shin with one or both hands.
- Stomp your standing heel into the ground and squeeze the glute of your standing leg without leaning your upper body back.
- Shift your same-side arm to the inside of the leg that's off the ground and grab your big toe with your first two fingers and your thumb.
- Kick your foot forward and extend your knee.

Variation

Standing Hand to Big Toe With Outward Hip Rotation

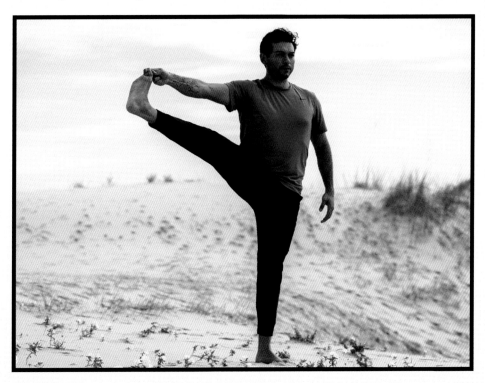

For more core and different leg activation, swing your leg out to the side while holding on to the big toe of the extended leg. Either keep your opposite arm down by your side (pictured) or extend it upward overhead. Activate the outer hip of the lifted leg to assist with the external rotation at the hip. Do not let your pelvis turn at an angle, but instead keep your hip bones squared off to the front of your space.

Standing Wide-Leg Forward Fold

Prasarita Padottanasana

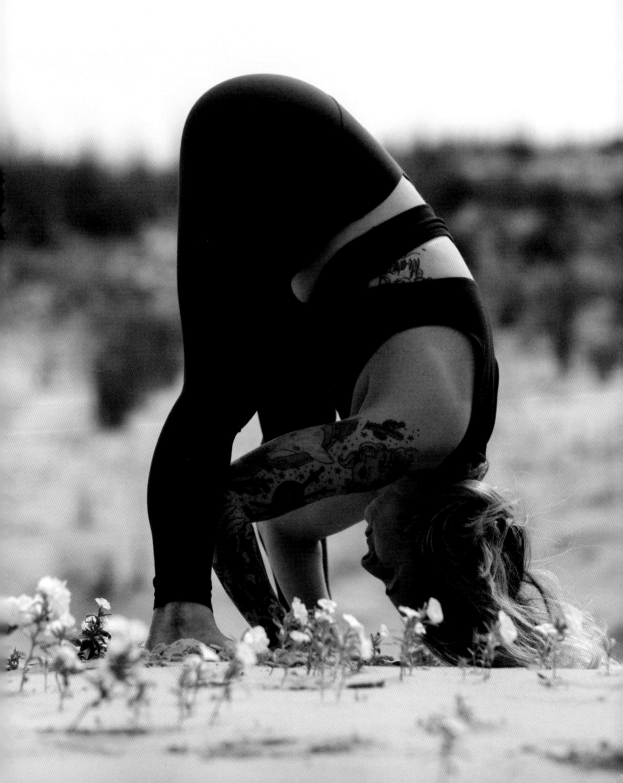

About This Pose

This standing forward fold strengthens the front of the legs and core while providing a deep stretch for the posterior chain. It is also an entry-level inversion and can be used as a transition to other inversions, such as headstand.

How To

- From mountain pose, place your hands on your hips and separate your feet significantly wider than hip-distance apart. Turn your feet so they are roughly parallel to each other.
- Hinge forward at your hips, maintaining the natural curve of your spine. Allow your weight to shift slightly back onto your heels without losing the contact of your entire foot on the floor and without locking your knees.
- When your spine is parallel with the ground—or you can no longer hinge with a neutral spine, whichever comes first—place your hands on the floor under your shoulders.
- Inhale and stretch the rib cage away from the hips.
- As you exhale, pull up your lower abdomen into the body to engage the lower core, engage the quadriceps, and contract the hip flexors to deepen the fold. Without locking your knees, balance your body weight equally over the heel and the ball of each foot.
- Allow your head to relax toward the floor, aiming the top of your skull between your feet.

Variation

Standing Wide-Leg Forward Fold With Arms Bound

From standing wide-leg forward fold, clasp your hands behind your back for shoulder extension and chest expansion. Reach your interlaced hands upward, away from your back, while rolling the tops of the shoulders (deltoid muscles and top of the humerus bones) toward your thoracic spine. Without your hands on the floor, it is even more tempting to lock the knees for balance; resist this temptation and continue to engage your quadriceps and core instead to find stability.

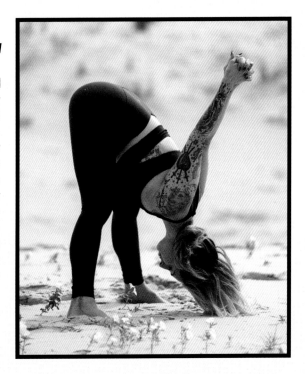

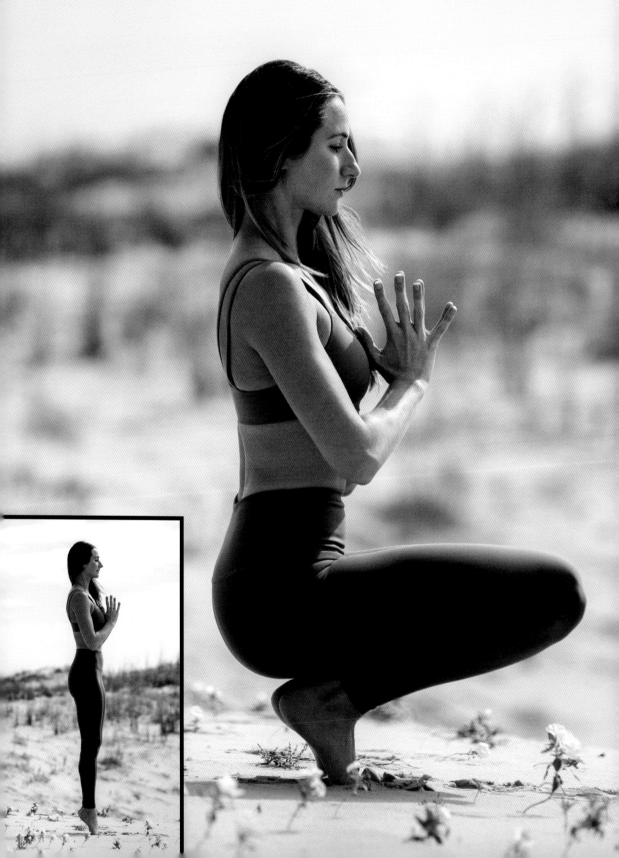

Toe Stand

Padangusthasana

About This Pose

Also called tiptoe, this pose can be deceptively challenging. It requires strength in the feet and ankles, quadriceps, and core to balance. Once you are comfortable practicing with both legs, you can try balancing on only one foot while lifting the other leg in front of you.

How To

- From mountain pose, lift your heels and balance on your tiptoes.
- Gaze at a stationary point several feet in front of you to assist your balancing efforts.
- Squeeze your legs together as you slowly bend your knees, and lower down until your hips hover over your heels.
- Align your head and shoulders over your hips and lower the knees so they are the same height as your hips. Your thighs will be parallel to the floor—but more important, you will feel the activation in your core rather than in the hip flexors.
- Lift your crown upward to lengthen the spine and hug the inner thighs together.

Variation

Toe Stand With Arm Extension

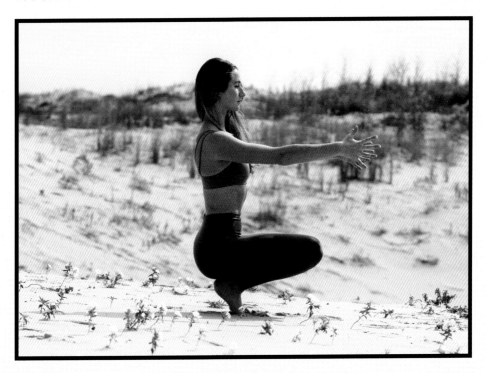

Experiment with arm variations. Hands in front of your body can act as a counterbalance for assistance, or take your arms overhead.

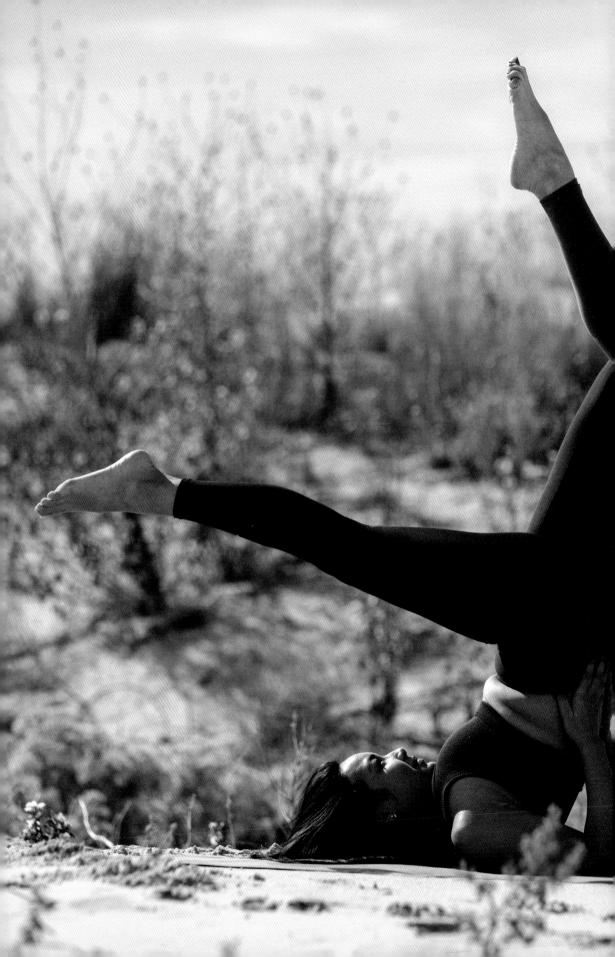

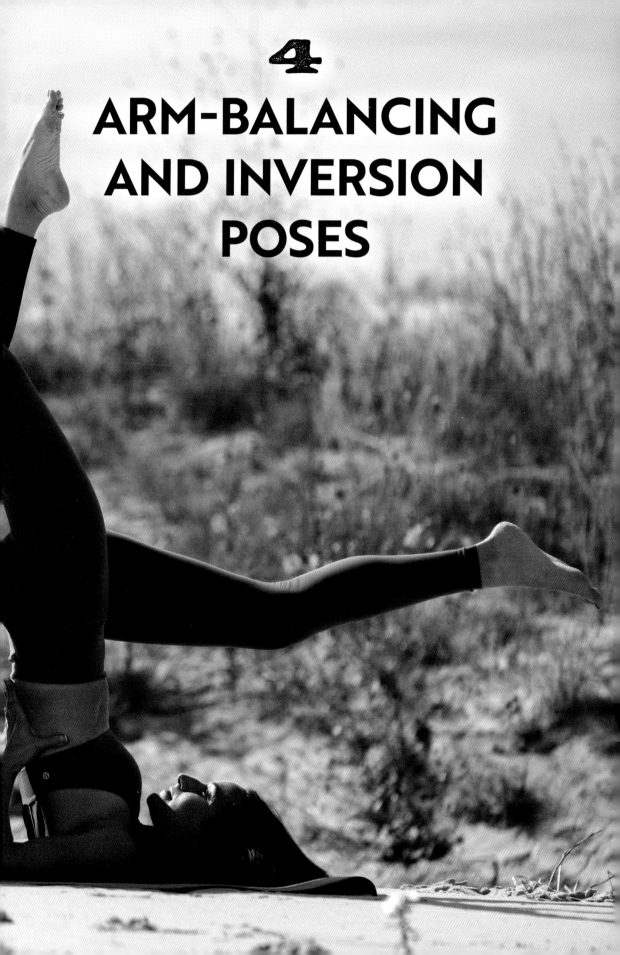

4

ARM-BALANCING AND INVERSION POSES

Crane/Crow
Bakasana/Kakasana

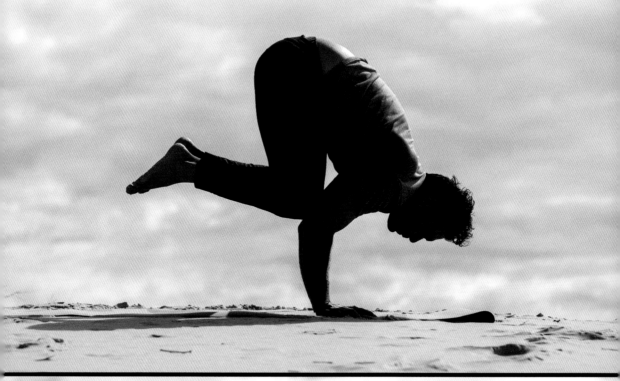

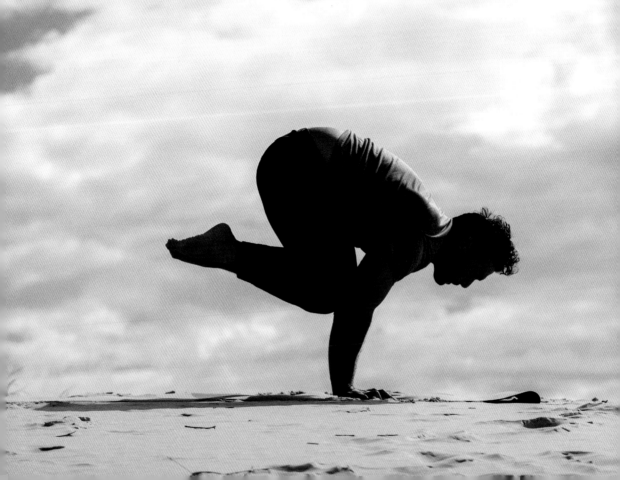

About This Pose

Bakasana (crane pose) or kakasana (crow pose) strengthens the core, arms, wrists, and hip flexors. In fact, many of the muscles that bring the body into flexion are used here—hamstrings, wrist flexors, pectoralis, and abdominals—to name a few. It is a foundational arm-balance and inversion posture because it not only introduces you to the strength requirements for your upper body, but it also balances your center of gravity and helps you face the fear of being upside down.

How To

- Place your hands on your mat roughly shoulder-width apart and grip the ground with your fingers; your fingers and how you grip will support your balance once your feet are off the floor.
- Place your knees on the backs of your upper arms.
- Squeeze everything into your center line and flex the spine as you engage your core, similar to cat pose. Focus on lifting your body upward from the ground and press downward with your hands, keeping the elbows bent between 45 to 90 degrees and pointing toward your heels.
- Without jutting your chin forward, lift your head to look forward at the ground while maintaining the natural curve in the back of your neck.
- Engage your hamstrings and lift your heels off the mat and toward your glutes.
- From crane, press downward into your hands and begin to straighten your arms as you continue to lift your body by engaging your core.

One-Legged Crow

Eka Pada Bakasana

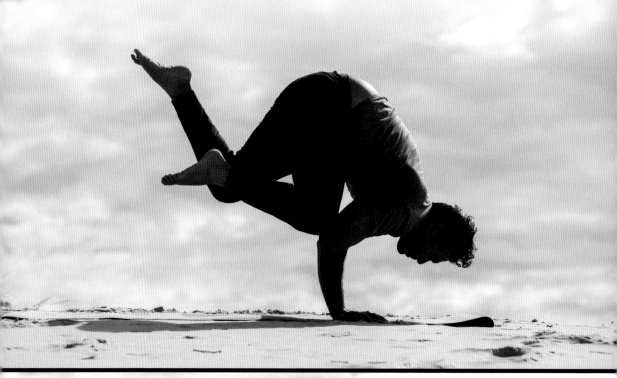

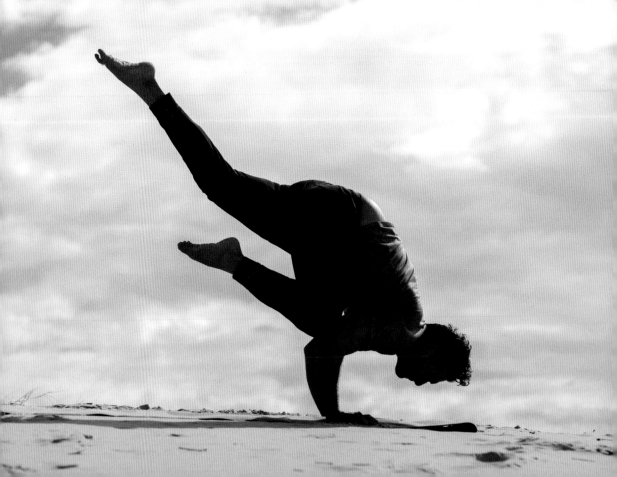

About This Pose

Similar to two-legged crow, this pose strengthens the core, arms, and wrists. An additional challenge for the core arises from the separate leg actions. I include two entrances into the pose because you may find one more approachable than the other based on your unique anatomy and strengths.

How To: Entrance One

- From a downward-facing dog pose, squeeze one knee tight into your armpit on the same side.
- Shift your weight forward and come onto the tiptoes of your back foot.
- Bend your elbows as you would in chaturanga dandasana so your center of gravity is more over your base (the hands). Push your upper arms against your knee and toward your hips to create strength and stability.
- Squeeze the glutes of your back leg to extend it up in the air, and then point your toes.

How To: Entrance Two

- From a forward fold position, place one knee on the back of your upper arm on the same side and bend your elbows as in a chaturanga dandasana pose.
- Shift your weight forward onto your hands and move your shoulders toward your hips to create strength and stability.
- Bring your opposite knee into your chest and engage the hamstring to lift your foot. Find your balance on your hands here in this small, tightly tucked position.
- Squeeze the glutes and quadriceps to extend the hip and send your elevated leg back and up behind you.

Side Crow

Parsva Bakasana

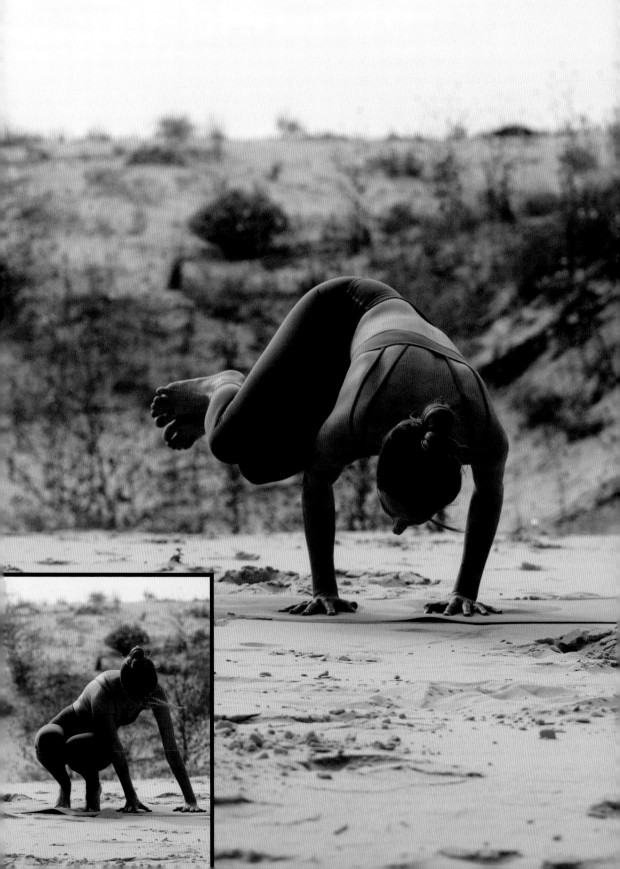

About This Pose

Side crow takes the low body position of crow and adds a deep twist through the spine. Because all of your weight is supported by one arm only, this pose also requires more upper-body strength.

How To

- From chair pose, twist your rib cage to the left side until you can hook your right arm on the outside of your left thigh.
- Reach down to place your right hand on the floor beside you, with your fingers pointing in the same direction as your toes. Note: This pose is sometimes taught in a way that turns your body 90 degrees. The instructions provided here naturally keep your hips higher, which takes less muscular effort than attempting to lift the hips up again while balancing.
- Aim to keep your hips as high as you can while you place your left hand on the floor. Notice that the hips do *not* rest on this arm.
- Squeeze your legs together and engage the lower core as you lean more onto your hands to lift your feet off the ground so your ankles squeeze together.
- Push your right arm against your legs to maintain shoulder stability as you use your obliques to rotate your rib cage to the right.

Variations

Side Crow With Straight Arms

Straighten the elbow that's not against your leg, or perhaps straighten both elbows. This involves a great amount of wrist extension, so make sure your wrists are healthy and strong; if not, avoid this pose.

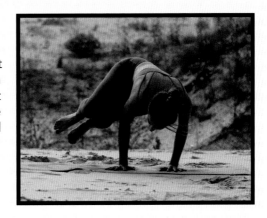

Side Crow With Straight Legs

Dwi Pada Koundinyasana

This is a straight-leg variation. Once your feet are lifted off the floor, squeeze the quadriceps and straighten your legs out to the side, above the ground.

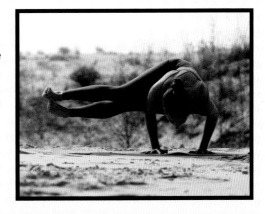

Hurdler

Dwi Pada Koundinyasana II

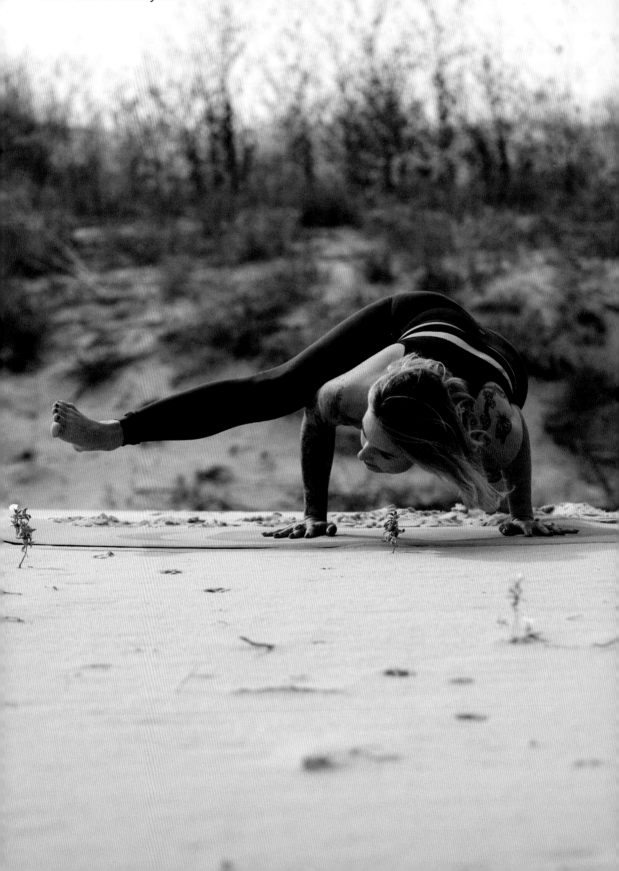

About This Pose

Like crow, this pose builds strength in the upper body—including the shoulders, biceps, and chest—as well as the core. Hurdler pose also requires hip mobility and hamstring stretching through the front leg.

How To

- From downward-facing dog, lift one leg up and back behind you, bend the knee, and open that hip out and slightly up.
- Bring your bent knee in toward the upper arm on the same side to squeeze your inner thigh to your outer triceps.
- With your knee pressed to the outside of your upper arm, bend your elbows (similar to four-limb staff pose) to create a shelf for your knee.
- Shift your weight forward and grip with your fingers as you lift your back leg off the ground, keeping the back leg extended straight back behind you.
- Extend your front leg and activate all 10 toes by flexing or pointing your feet.

Eight-Angle Pose

Astavakrasana

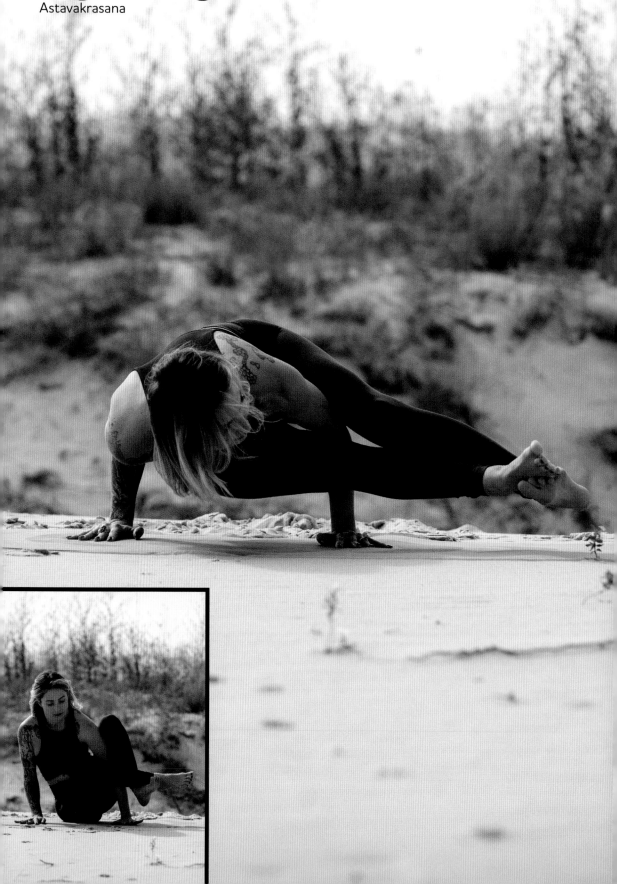

About This Pose

Like all arm balances, this pose requires solid strength in the legs and core to support the upper-body effort in the wrists, arms, and shoulders. In addition, astavakrasana stretches the back of the legs and hips while twisting the spine. Because you can enter this pose from a seated position, you may find it more accessible and less intimidating than some of the other arm-balancing poses.

How To

- From seated staff position, use your hands to hook your left leg over your left shoulder from behind your back like a backpack strap. If the leg doesn't get all the way to the shoulder, that's okay! It can rest on the upper arm.
- Place your hands on either side of your thighs about midway between your hips and your knees. This forward position will come in handy for the arm balance.
- Hook your right ankle on top of the left ankle of your lifted leg. Squeeze your inner thighs around your upper arm and engage the quadriceps to extend the knees.
- As you lean forward and bend your elbows, hollow out the lower belly and lift your hips up.
- Engage your serratus and latissimus muscles under your shoulders by pushing your hands down and forward as you move your chest forward toward the floor.

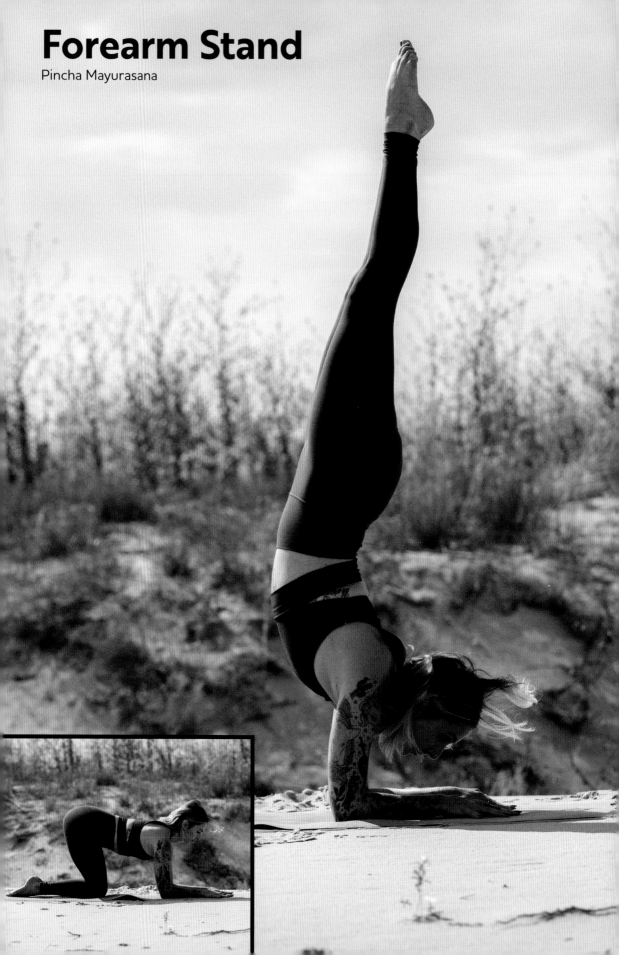

Forearm Stand
Pincha Mayurasana

About This Pose

This pose resembles handstand except rather than balancing on your wrists, you support your weight on your forearms. Even with the broader base, this pose can sometimes be more challenging because your elbows and wrists cannot make up for any lack of shoulder mobility and there is less opportunity to balance and counterbalance.

How To

- In a kneeling position sitting on your shins, place your forearms on the floor parallel to one another and roughly shoulder-distance apart, with either the pinky sides or the palms of your hands on the ground.
- Tuck your toes and lift your knees off the mat to move your hips high in the air.
- Lift up onto your tiptoes and carefully walk your feet toward your elbows. This will move your hips over the base created by your shoulders.
- Extend one leg straight up in the air and lean your weight forward onto your arms as much as possible.
- Keeping the core engaged, push through the ground and lift your second leg up to meet the first. Squeeze your legs toward your midline.
- Push down to the ground and reach up through your feet. Gaze between your forearms.

Flying Pigeon
Eka Pada Galavasana

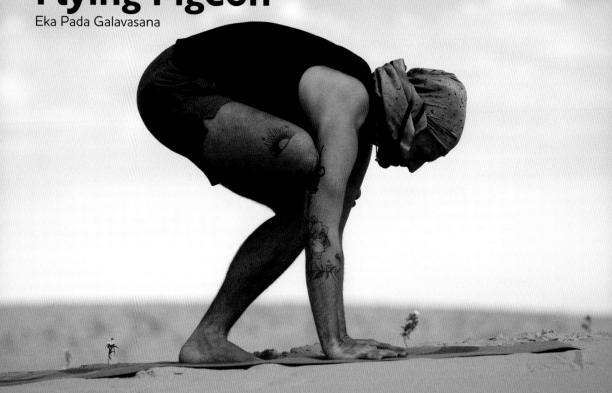

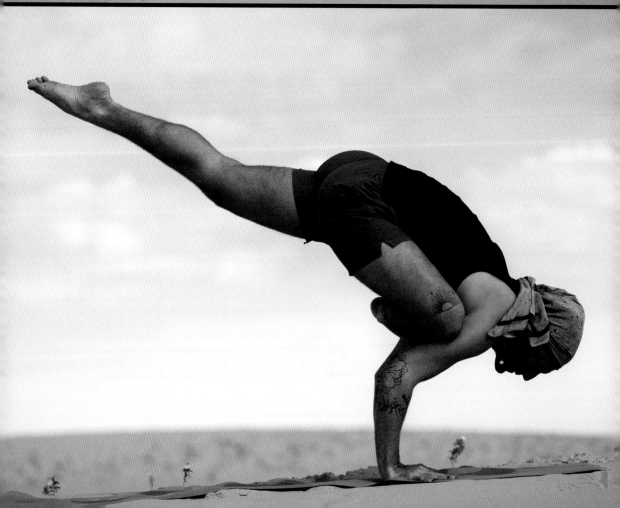

About This Pose

Like many arm balances, this pose requires strength in the arms, shoulders, and core. It also requires quite a bit of external hip rotation of your front leg. The leg setup resembles one-legged king pigeon but in a more active stretch variation as you kick your legs in opposite directions to fly.

How To

- From chair pose, cross your right ankle over your left knee in a figure four. Place your hands on the ground in front of you and press your right shin into your upper arms. Grip your left upper arm with the toes of your right foot.
- Bend forward and place your hands on the floor in front of you roughly shoulder-distance apart. As you lean forward onto your hands, bend your elbows like chaturanga dandasana to create a shelf for your lower body. Push your arms against your right leg to stabilize the shoulders.
- Grip the ground with your fingers and press down through your knuckles as they become your brakes.
- Once you find your balance, engage your left hamstring to bring your foot off the ground.
- Keep the lower core engaged. Squeeze your glutes and extend your left leg back and up behind you. There is an equal and opposite lengthening action—your front leg kicks forward into your arms while you stretch out through the back leg.

Handstand
Adho Mukha Vrksasana

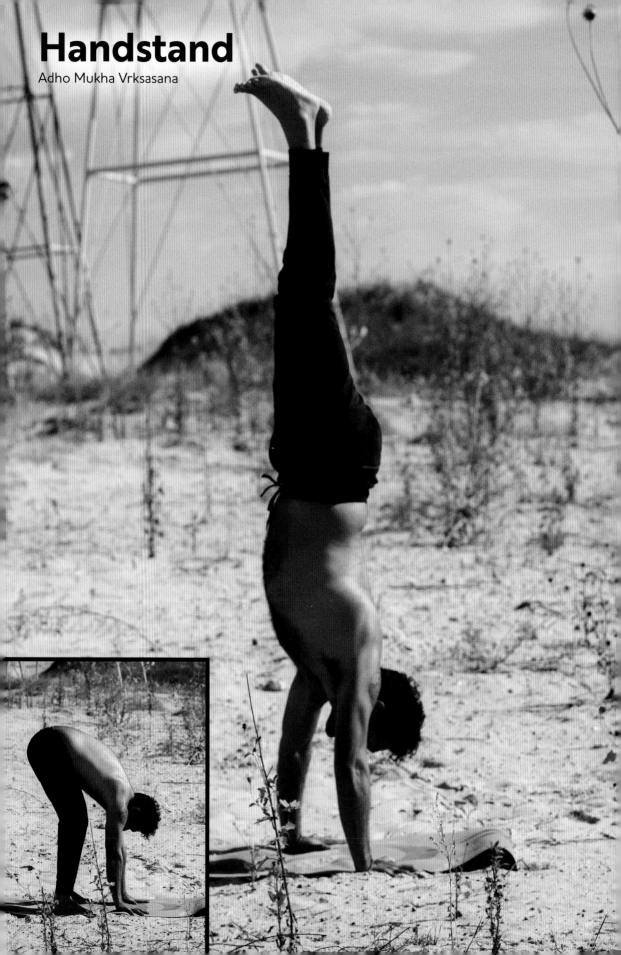

About This Pose

This classic arm balance requires strength, stability, and awareness in the entire body, like many arm balances. However, this pose also requires a higher level of strength at the end range of shoulder flexion. There are so many different perspectives and variations on the handstand. This entrance is foundational to learn before moving on to more advanced versions. The separate-leg position allows you to experience under- and overbalance so you can spend more time building endurance upside down.

How To

- From a standing position, bend forward and place your hands on the mat shoulder-width apart. Spread your fingers wide because they will act as your brakes when you're balancing.
- Walk your feet forward until your shoulders are aligned over your wrists. Lift your heels and bend your knees as needed to lift your hips higher.
- Send one leg up straight and strong and as high as you can. Lift onto the tiptoes of your standing foot and take little hops until you feel your hips balance over the base of support in your hands.
- Use this split-leg position to balance and counterbalance as you learn to be comfortable pushing into the ground and being upside down.
- Push your hands into the floor rather than allowing your weight to sink onto your shoulders and wrists.
- Gaze between your wrists.
- When your balance is steady, slowly bring the legs together. Engage all the muscles in your legs and squeeze the inner thighs together as you reach up through your feet.

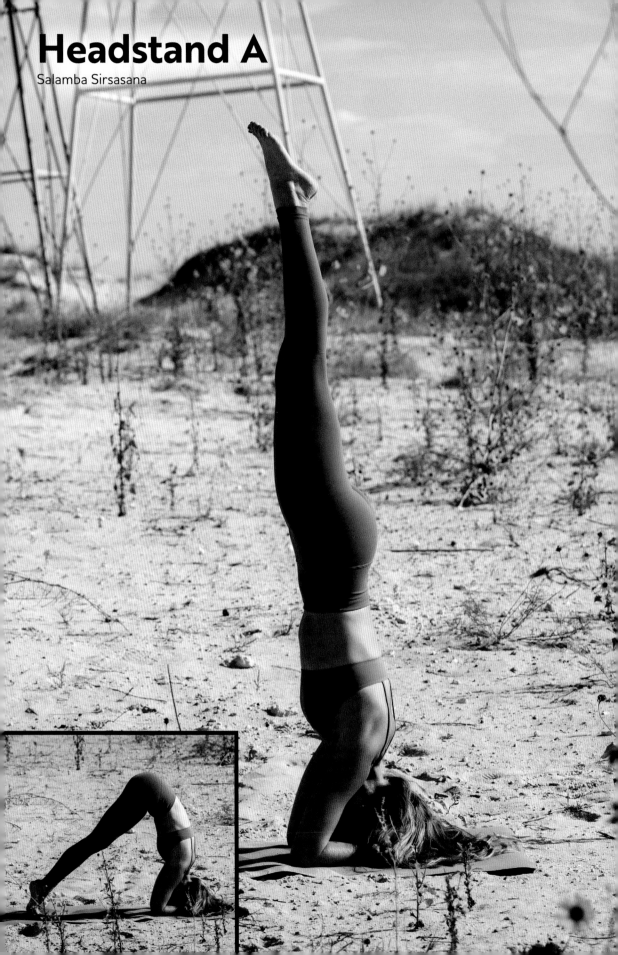

Headstand A
Salamba Sirsasana

About This Pose

Headstand is considered by some to be the king of all poses. Although that is highly debatable, headstand is a fantastic inversion for your yoga journey. It builds strength in the shoulders, core, and legs while providing all the circulatory and mental benefits of inversions. This variation on headstand is one of the most supported, so there is less weight on your head and neck. While many students learn this pose first for that reason, the foundation of the arms is quite constricted. Broad-shouldered or short-limbed yogis may find this pose more difficult to set up and will have more success with tripod headstand (headstand B).

How To

- From tabletop, lower your elbows to the floor directly under your shoulders. Interlace your fingers, leaving a small space between your palms. Your elbows and hands will form something close to an equilateral triangle as your base.
- Place the top of your head on the floor between your hands so your hands cup the back of your head.
- Push your elbows and wrists into the ground to stabilize the shoulders as you lift your knees to move your hips up.
- Walk your feet toward your face as far as you can to move the hips over the base of your head and arms.
- Carefully lift both feet off the floor and hug your thighs toward your belly to compress the front of your hips. Depending on your hamstring and hip flexibility, this can be done with straight or bent knees.
- Slowly extend your legs straight into the air until your feet are over your hips and your hips are over your shoulders and head. Continuously press down into the floor with your forearms and stretch up and out through the feet. Engage the deep core as you breathe steadily.
- To focus your mind and assist in finding balance, gaze at a stationary spot a few feet in front of you.
- To exit the pose, bend your knees to place your feet on the floor and lower to tabletop or child's pose.

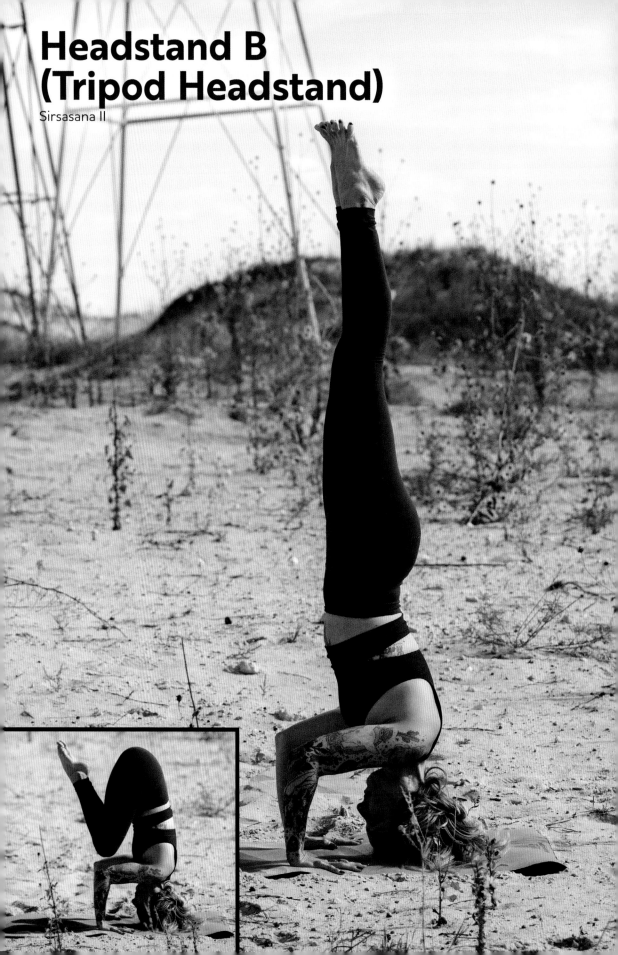

Headstand B
(Tripod Headstand)
Sirsasana II

About This Pose

This headstand variation has a base with less support and assistance from the arms. However, depending on your shoulder anatomy and mobility, it can feel more accessible. In ashtanga and other flow styles, this headstand is not held for long but used as a transition between arm-balancing poses. It is common to set up your tripod base incorrectly, with the head too close to the hands, which decreases the stability and strength in your shoulders. Visualize the triangle of your head (top of the triangle) and hands (base of the triangle) before placing your head down because making adjustments once you have weight on your head is precarious.

How To

- From tabletop, tuck your chin and place the top of your head on the floor in front of your hands to form an equilateral triangle. Your elbows align over your hands and create 90-degree angles at the wrists, elbows, and shoulders.
- Hug your elbows in toward each other to activate your pectorals as you push both hands and your head firmly into the floor. Gaze at a nonmoving point a few feet away to help with balance.
- One at a time, bring a knee into your chest and place it onto the same-side elbow. Once you are stable being upside down, strongly engage the core and lift both knees off your arms to create a tuck position.
- Slowly extend both legs upward, keeping the muscles tight and hugging into your midline from all sides.
- A progression of the entrance would be to keep both legs straight and lift them together without resting your knees on your arms.

Shoulder Stand
Salamba Sarvangasana

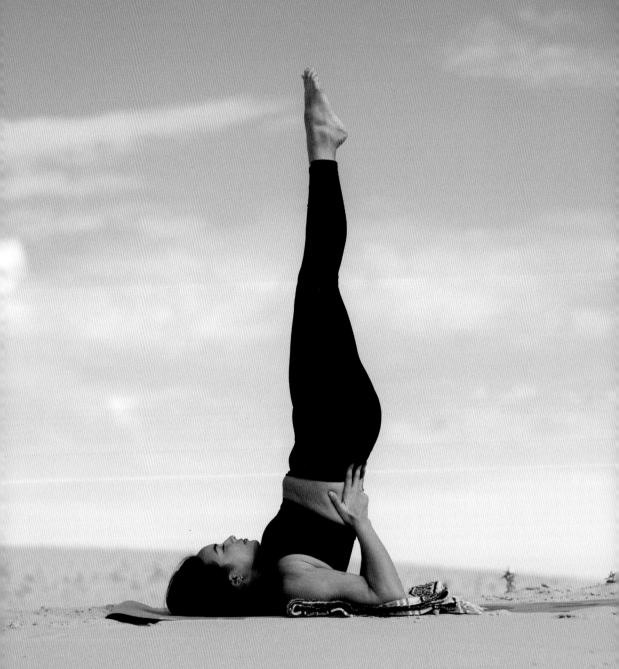

About This Pose

Shoulder stand is considered more restorative than other inversions because the balance challenge is considerably less, and it can be more accessible to newer yogis. However, I would not consider it a beginner pose because the subtle details in the setup are crucial to the safety of the pose and the neck is in a precarious position. Like all inversions, this pose strengthens your legs and core while encouraging blood and lymph circulation.

How To

- Stack several yoga mats or firm blankets so you have a minimum 1-inch (2.5 cm) height. Lie down with your shoulders at the end of the props, with your head on the floor. This setup will reduce the strain on the delicate muscles of your neck.
- With your arms by your sides, line up your heels in front of your sitz bones, with your knees pointing upward, and engage the muscles of your legs and activate the deep core.
- Push your arms into the floor as you use your core and hip flexors to swing your straight legs and hips up in the air.
- Bend your elbows and place your hands on your lower back. Slowly walk your hands up your back toward your shoulders and move your chest toward your chin.
- Extend your legs and lift your feet in alignment over your hips and shoulders. Keep the core and glutes engaged as you press your shoulders into the floor and squeeze your elbows toward one another.
- To come out of the pose, bend at the hips so your feet move past your head. Slowly roll down—upper back, middle back, lower back, then hips. Bend your knees to plant your feet on the floor.

Ear-Pressing Pose

Karnapidasana

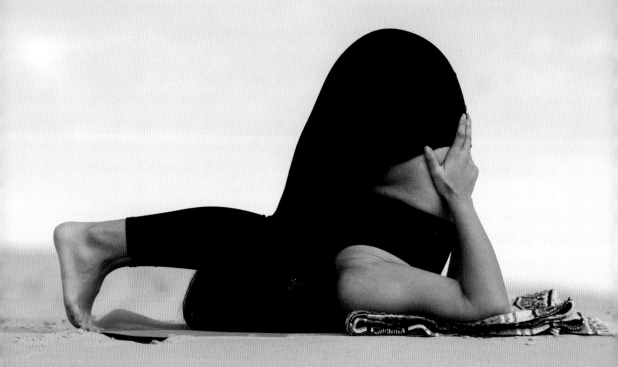

About This Pose

This inversion commonly appears before or after shoulder stand and has numerous benefits. It stretches all the spinal extensors used for backbends and for staying upright throughout the day, as well as the back of the hips and legs. It can improve the movement of the bottom half of the rib cage during respiration. Many people find these restorative inversions to be quite calming on the nervous system.

How To

- Stack several yoga mats or firm blankets so you have minimum 1-inch (2.5 cm) height. Lie down with your shoulders at the end of the props, with your head on the floor. This setup will reduce the strain on the delicate muscles of your neck.
- With your arms by your sides, engage the muscles of your legs and activate the deep core. Walk your feet up to your hips so that your feet are on the mat and your knees are pointing upward.
- Push your arms into the floor as you use your core and hip flexors to swing your straight legs and hips up until your feet find the floor over your head.
- Bend your elbows to take your hands to your back. Slowly walk your hands up your back toward your shoulders and move your chest toward your chin. Keep your hands supporting your back (pictured) or straighten your elbows and interlace your fingers. Push your arms into the floor for stability and shoulder strength.
- Bend your knees and lower them to the floor beside your ears. Gently press your knees to your ears.
- Actively squeeze your thighs toward your spine and your spine toward your thighs.

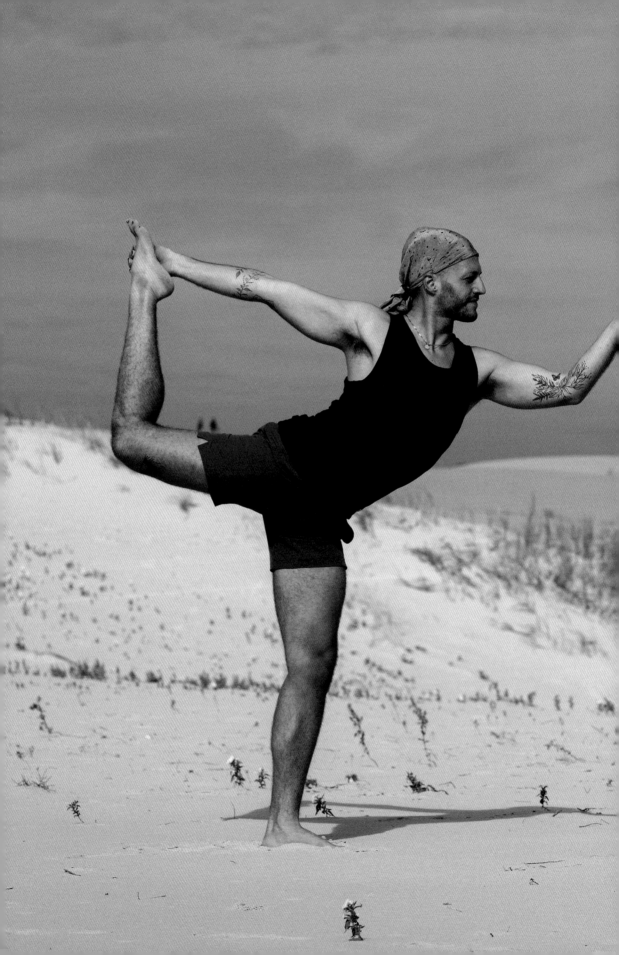

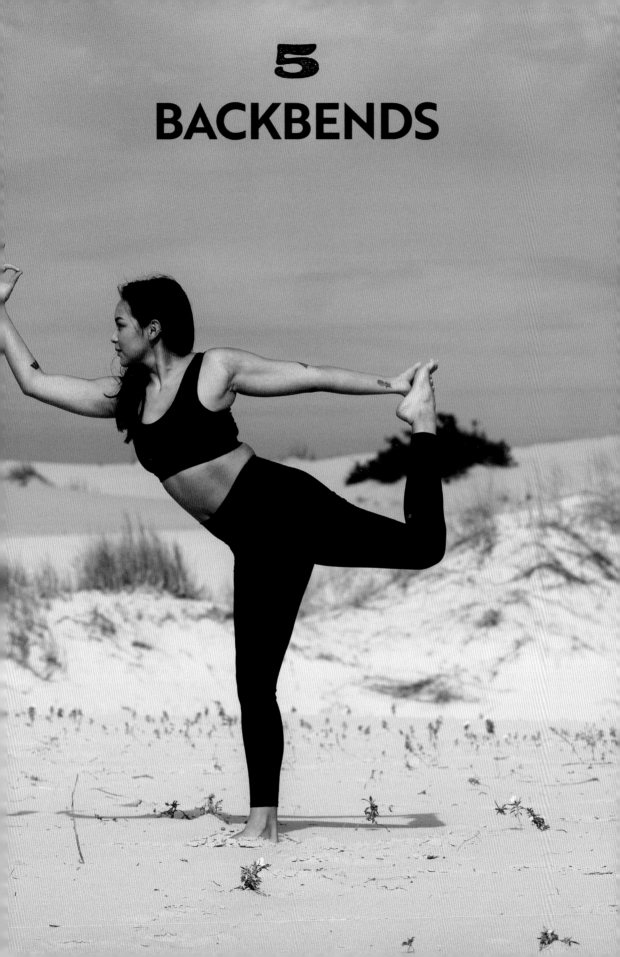

5
BACKBENDS

Upward-Facing Dog

Urdhva Mukha Svanasana

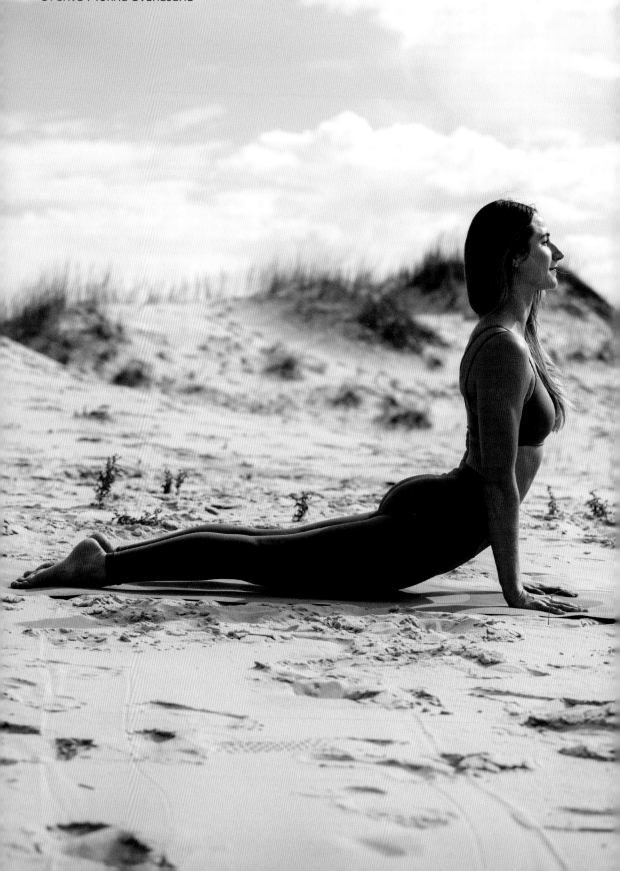

About This Pose

Upward-facing dog is the standard backbend of the modern sun salutation sequence. However, just because it is standard and used many times, does *not* mean it is easy! It requires balancing on the hands and the feet, and it strengthens both the upper and lower body. While it can be tempting to relax into the backbend and allow gravity to do the work, use your back muscles to deepen the backbend. This will create a strong and sustainable pose.

How To

- Lie face down, with your legs extended and the tops of your feet on the ground.
- Place your hands alongside your ribs so that your elbows bend roughly 90 degrees.
- Retract and press your shoulder blades together on your back and down toward your hips.
- Squeeze the glutes and push the tops of your feet into the ground so your legs are engaged.
- Push the ground away with your hands to lift your chest. Energetically drag your arms back toward your feet to pull your chest forward and coil upward until your pelvis lifts off the ground.
- Gently move your head back to bring the chin toward the chest—so you give yourself a slight double chin—before looking up and slightly back.

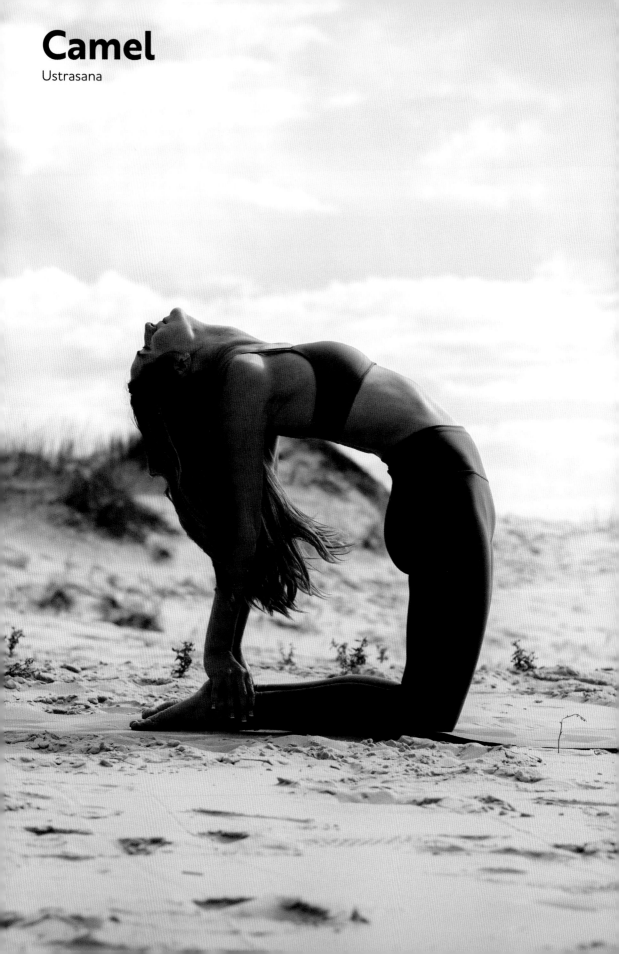

Camel
Ustrasana

About This Pose

Camel is similar in shape to bridge pose, yet because of the relationship to gravity, you can experience the effort of the pose quite differently. This pose requires strong work in the legs and core without the leverage of pushing down into the ground through your feet. Gravity will assist your backbend initially as you bend backward, so you must use your back muscles and mental focus to continuously lift the chest up. This will lessen the compression in your lower back and create even more expansion in the front of the body.

How To

- Kneel on your shins with your legs roughly hip-distance apart.
- Move your inner thighs toward each other and engage the deep core as you squeeze your glutes.
- Inhale and lengthen your rib cage up away from your hips.
- Exhale and bend backward, maintaining length in the spine, until your hands touch your heels.
- Push your hands down into your heels and squeeze your shoulder blades together on your back to lift your chest upward.
- Tuck your chin toward the chest—so you have a slight double chin—before gently dropping your head back. Gaze up or behind without straining your neck.

Bow
Dhanurasana

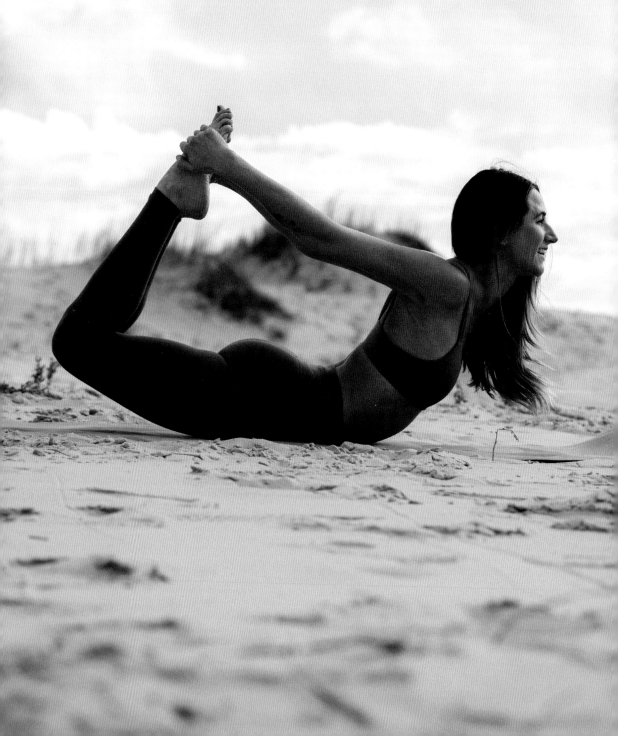

About This Pose

Dhanurasana is a prone backbend where you are working against gravity to lift yourself up. Without the assistance of your arms or legs to push into the ground, this pose requires tremendous strength in the posterior chain, particularly the glutes and extensors of the back. The contracting of the back side of the body provides a deep stretch for your entire front side, especially the hip flexors, abdominals, and chest.

How To

- Lying face down, bend your knees and reach your hands back to grab your ankles or feet.
- Kick your feet into your hands to lift your chest away from the floor.
- Squeeze your glutes, particularly where your glutes and hamstrings meet; this will prevent your knees from splaying wider than your hips. Push your feet upward to extend the hips and lift your thigh bones off the floor.
- Even though your legs can help power the backbend, engage the muscles in your back to actively stretch your chest.

Variation

Unbound Bow

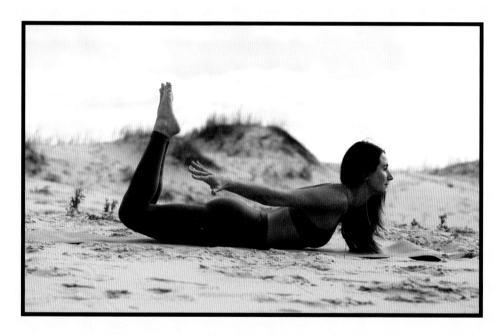

Rather than gripping your legs with your hands, hover your hands next to your legs. This will build even more strength in the posterior chain, especially the hamstrings and erector spinae muscles of the back.

Upward-Facing Bow

Urdhva Dhanurasana

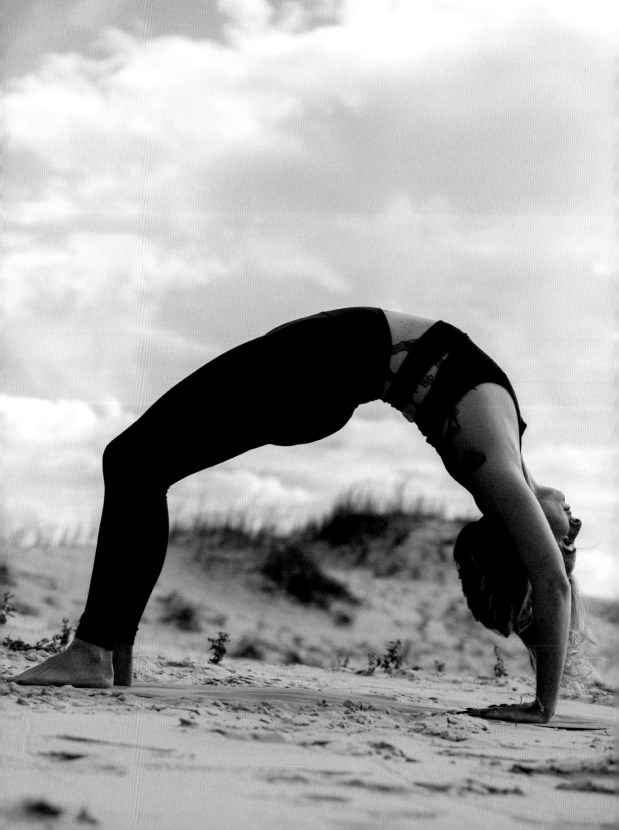

About This Pose

The name "upward-facing bow" (also commonly known as wheel) implies similarities to bow, and it does in fact appear to be bow pose flipped upside down. However, considering that the effort of the pose is mostly spent resisting gravity, the sensations felt will often not be the same initially. Once you have pushed up into the pose, many similar muscle activations—contracting the posterior chain—take place to deepen the backbend in a sustainable way.

How To

- Lying on your back, bend your knees and place your feet flat on the mat. Reach down and check that you can graze your ankles with your fingertips. This will ensure your feet are more underneath your legs and give you more leverage to push into the ground.
- Place your hands on either side of your head, wider than your shoulders. Your options are to turn your fingers toward your feet or face them out to the sides, which is more accessible. Also, widen your hands apart to accommodate your shoulder mobility and flexibility.
- On an exhale, engage the deep core and glutes to create a slight posterior tilt of the pelvis. You will have more access to this action here as opposed to when you are already in the backbend.
- Push the ground away with your hands and feet to lift your hips and shoulders into the air.
- As you push your heels down, isometrically drag them toward your hands to engage the hamstrings and glutes. Keep the deep core engaged so there is a sensation of your pubic bone moving higher and toward your rib cage. Put another way: Attempt to lift the bottom of your pelvis at your pubic bone more than you lift your hip bones.
- Retract the shoulder blades more onto your back as you press your chest past your arms.
- Breathe in as you lengthen your chest and knees in opposite directions. You are not simply lifting up but stretching the entire front of your body.

Variations

One-Leg Upward-Facing Bow

Eka Pada Urdhva Dhanurasana

Walk one foot more to the center of your mat as you bring your opposite knee to your chest. Squeeze the quadriceps and extend your foot in the air.

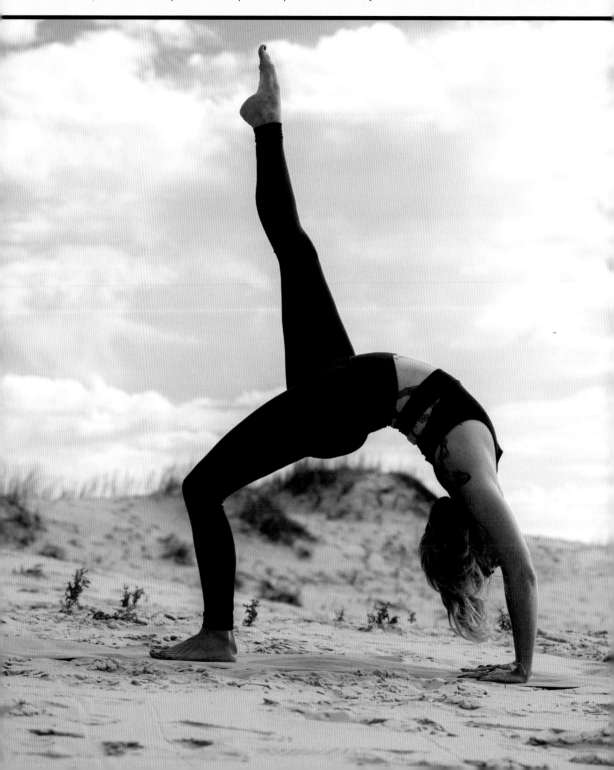

Forearm Wheel

From upward-facing bow, lower from your hands to your forearms and interlace your fingers behind your head. Walk your feet forward to straighten your legs while maintaining the lift of the front of your body. Press your feet into the mat and engage your legs. Reach your chest in the opposite direction of your feet to find more extension in the mid and upper back.

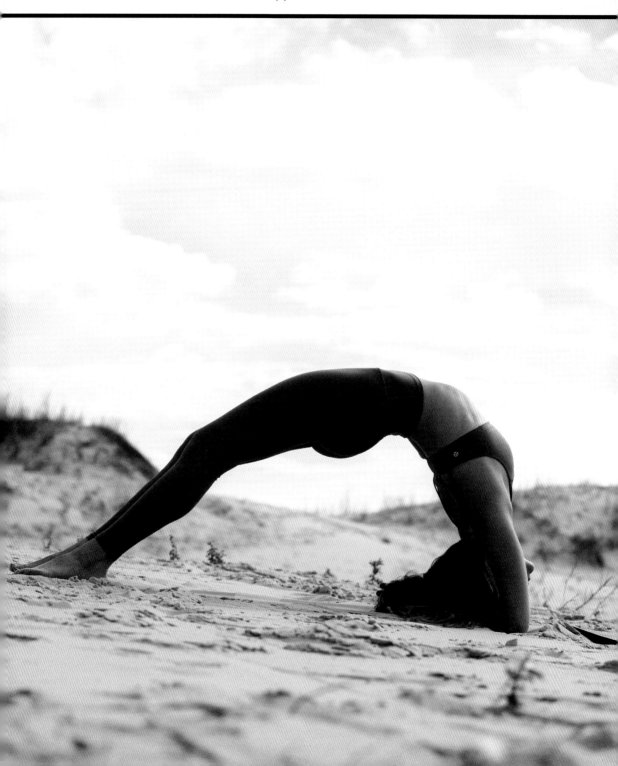

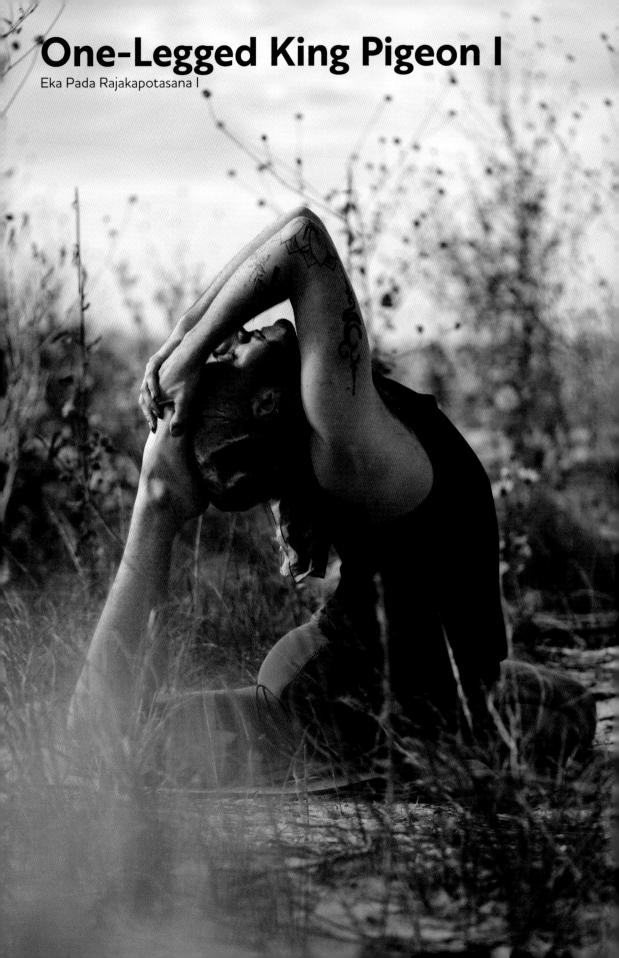

One-Legged King Pigeon I

Eka Pada Rajakapotasana I

About This Pose

This challenging pose requires not only deep flexibility of the front hip but also of the hip flexors of the rear leg and the front of the torso to create a deep backbend. Many modern classes eliminate the backbend in this pose and instruct you to fold forward to rest your chest and head on the ground. With our modern lifestyles of sitting in cars, at our computers, and in front of the television, I like to balance the folded variation with the upright variations described here to stretch the front of the body and strengthen both the back of the body and the core.

How To

- From an easy, seated, cross-leg position, swing one leg behind you. Your front thigh is externally rotated, with your knee wider than your hip and your foot roughly in front of your opposite hip. Keeping the knee in deep flexion—heel closer to the hip—will prevent extraneous twisting in the knee.
- Breathe in to expand your ribs and lift them away from your hips.
- Bend your back knee and grab hold of your foot with the same-side hand. Engage your deep core, pelvic floor, and glutes to stabilize through your center and find balance.
- Reach your opposite arm overhead, bend the elbow, and grab your back foot.
- Release the grip of your same-side hand in order to reach that arm overhead, then bend the elbow and grasp your foot now with both hands.
- Even though gravity and the pose itself will move you closer to the ground, energetically hug your legs and deep core in and up to create space for the backbend as well as stability in the hips.
- Continue to lift your rib cage up as you find full extension of the spine and your head touches your foot.

Variation

One-Legged King Pigeon I Upright Without a Bind

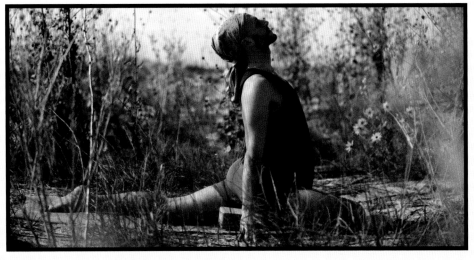

Support one or both hips with a bolster, pillow, or block and use your hands to assist the lift of your chest.

One-Legged King Pigeon II

Eka Pada Rajakapotasana II

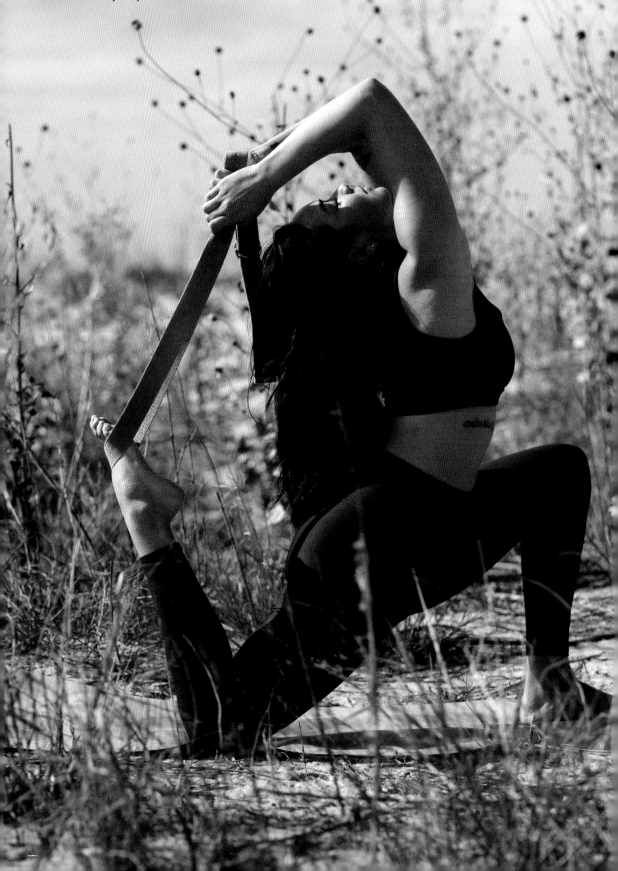

About This Pose

This variation on one-legged king pigeon changes the position of the front leg from deep external rotation to a lunge. Although some yogis will find this to be more challenging than the first variation, others actually find this pose to be more stable and accessible. The lengthening demands on the hip flexor of the back leg are much more obvious in this elevated position; however, the front foot on the ground offers more strength and assistance to lift up and create the backbend. Once again, your unique anatomy and flexibility will determine what it feels like and looks like.

How To

- In a crescent low lunge, or anjaneyasana, position your front foot a couple inches out to the side and past your hip. Engage the core and the glute of the back leg as you shift your pelvis forward and down to deepen the hip flexor stretch. Try not to rush this because it is the foundation for your backbend.
- Breathe in to expand your ribs and lift them away from your hips.
- Bend your back knee in toward your hip by activating your hamstring as if you are doing a hamstring curl. Grab hold of your back foot with your same-side hand or use a strap to grab your foot if you cannot reach with your hand. Engage your deep core, pelvic floor, and glutes to stabilize through your center and find balance.
- Reach your opposite arm overhead, bend the elbow, and grab your back foot or grab the strap if you are using one.
- Release the grip of the same-side hand from your foot or strap in order to reach that arm overhead. Bend the elbow and grasp your foot or strap now with both hands.
- Tuck your pelvis using the glutes and core muscles as you press your front foot into the floor and slightly lift the hips and rib cage. Many times, the instinct is to sink low for a deeper bend, but lifting up and back will actually give you access to the full shape.
- Continue to lift your rib cage up as you find full extension of the spine, drawing your head and foot toward each other using the strap.
- Gaze up and slightly back or close your eyes.

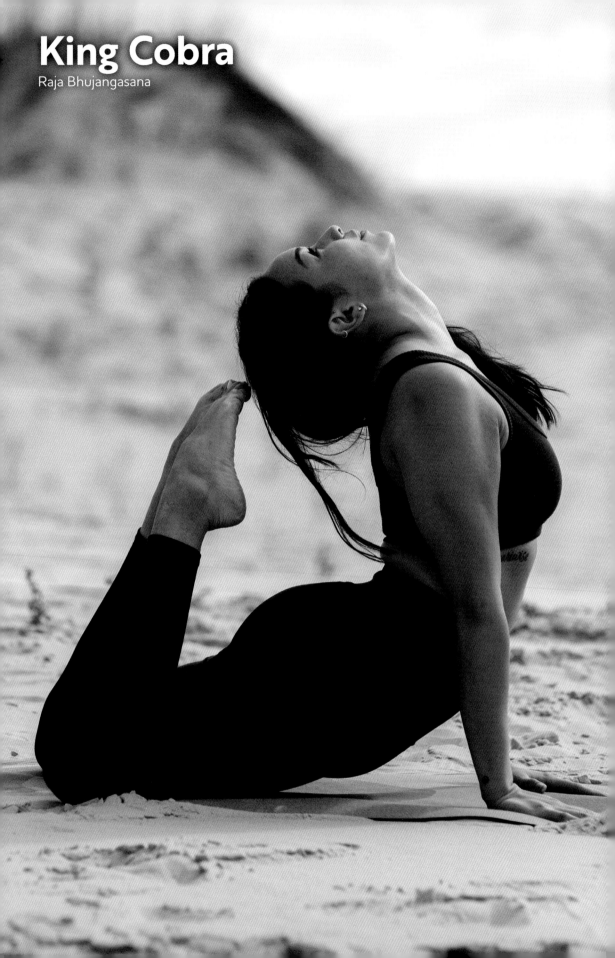

King Cobra

Raja Bhujangasana

About This Pose

This challenging pose requires contracting the entire posterior chain against gravity. Bear in mind that the length of your legs relative to your spine, as well as the mobility of your legs and spine, will cause the exact shape to vary compared with that of another practitioner. The goal is to actively extend throughout the spine, extend the hips, and flex the knees to intensely stretch the front of the body.

How To

- From upward-facing dog, drop your thighs and pubic bone to the floor.
- Lift your palms so that only your fingertips touch the ground. This will elevate your torso by several inches and create more working space in the pose.
- Inhale and elevate the rib cage up and out from the hips, creating length in the spine.
- Squeeze the glutes and engage the hamstrings to bend both knees. Point your toes.
- Move your head straight back as you tuck your chin toward the chest, giving yourself a slight double chin, before gently dropping your head back.
- Repeat the pattern of inhaling to create length and lift and exhaling to bend deeper into the pose.
- Even though the lumbar spine is in extension, engage the glutes and deep core above the pubic bone (as if you could posteriorly tuck your pelvis) and flex the spine.

Dancer
Natarajasana

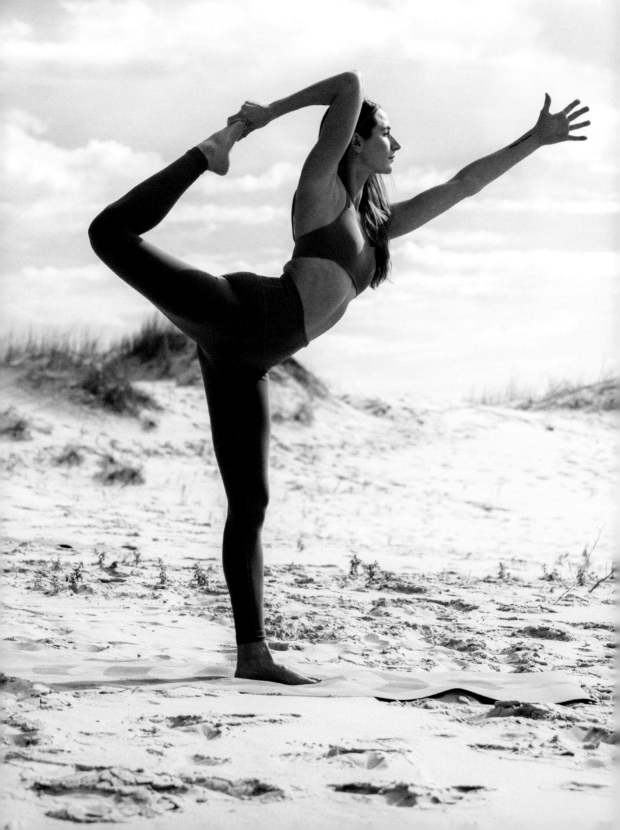

About This Pose

Dancer requires not just a strong backbend of the spine similar to one-legged king pigeon or king cobra but also adds the challenge of balancing on one leg. Two common variations involve either grabbing the foot with both hands—increasing the demands on your shoulder mobility—or lessening the demands by holding the lifted foot back behind the torso without flipping the grip and extending the elbow overhead.

How To

- From mountain pose, shift your weight to one leg as you reach the same-side arm upward.
- With your opposite arm down by your thigh, externally rotate your entire arm so that your biceps and palm face outward.
- Bend your knee and grab hold of your foot with this hand. Your fingers will grip the pinky-toe side of your foot and your thumb should point up. Yes, it is an awkward grip when you are new to the pose, but it will make the transition of your arm overhead much more accessible.
- During this phase of setup, it is helpful to bend your knee. Not only will this allow you more freedom to bend, but it also encourages more muscle engagement in the standing leg. You will create more strength and balance at the same time.
- Lift the foot off the ground close to the hip so that your elbow can bend and your arm is not fully extended behind you. Extend your elbow out to the side and overhead to position the arm for the final pose.
- To encourage your chest to lift, reach your free arm up on a diagonal at whatever angle your mobility allows.
- Squeeze the glutes to extend your back foot upward, keeping your chest high.
- Engage the quadriceps of your standing leg and lift the deep core away from the floor.

Fish
Matsyasana

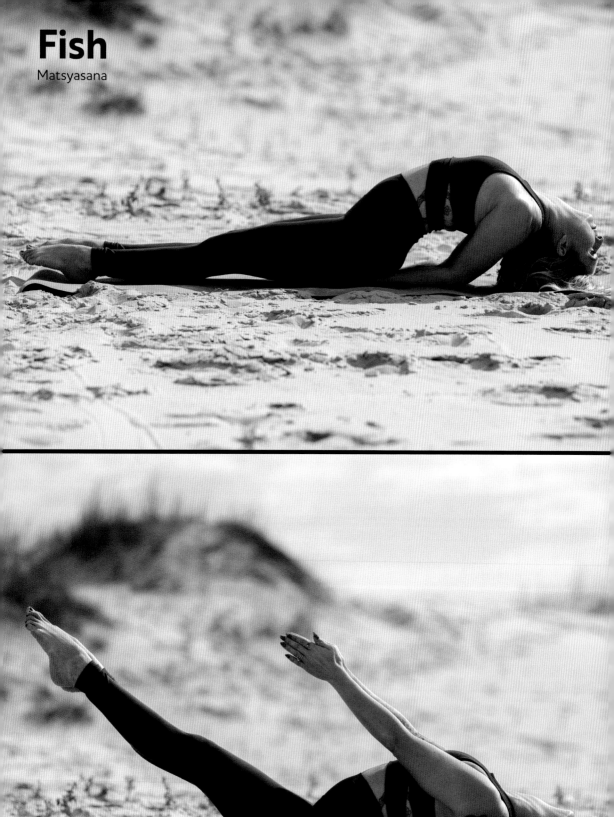

About This Pose

Matsyasana is a backbend that uses shoulder extension and hip flexion to strengthen many of the muscles that get less attention in yoga practice. This pose is an extension for the spine, but unlike many other backbends, it involves flexion at the hips. This increases the need for stability in the deep core to avoid straining the hip flexors, including the psoas. Combined with the positioning of the arms and pushing against the floor, this pose can often feel constrictive—you might not experience this backbend as free or invigorating as some others.

How To

- Lying on your back, tuck your elbows under your shoulders so that your upper arms are roughly vertical and your forearms are parallel.
- Push your hands and elbows into the ground as you squeeze your shoulder blades together on your back. Inhale to expand your front rib cage.
- Move your head forward to tuck the chin toward the chest, giving yourself a slight double chin, before gently dropping your head back. There should not be immense pressure on your head.
- Point your toes and engage your quadriceps so your legs are straight and knees are tight.
- Exhale and engage the deep core to hollow out the lower belly and avoid doming in the abdominals.
- Keep your legs strong and straight and lift them as high as you can. Try to close the space between your front hip bones and upper thighs. If your abdominals dome outward or you feel strain in the lower back, practice with your legs on the ground.
- Continuously push your arms down and engage your back muscles, bringing your shoulder blades together and toward your hips to expand the chest.
- If your head is on the ground with very light pressure on the top of the skull, you can reach your arms in front of your chest with the palms pressing together. This requires strong engagement of the erector spinae to hold yourself up without collapsing onto your head and putting pressure on your neck.

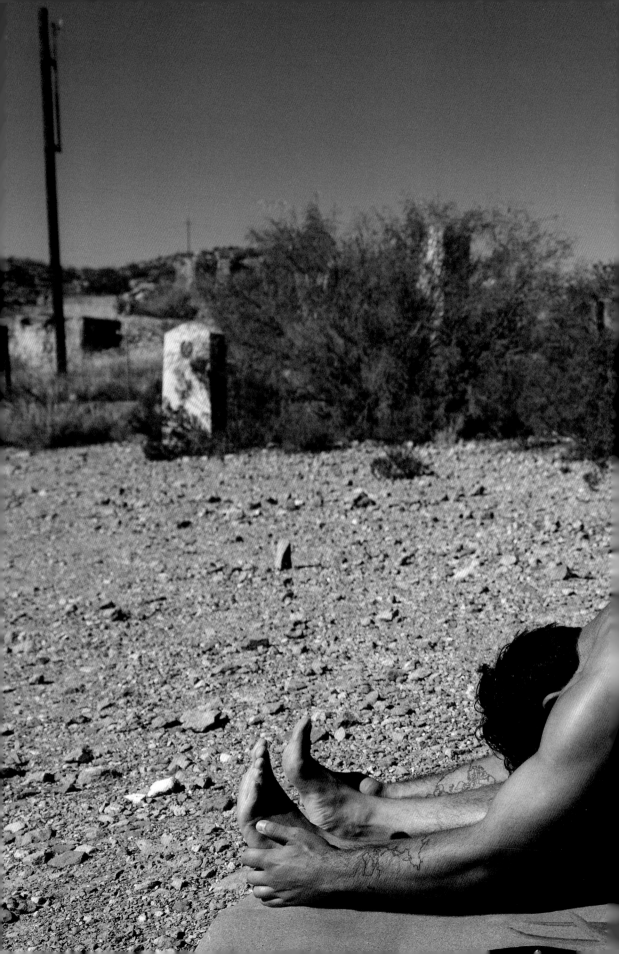

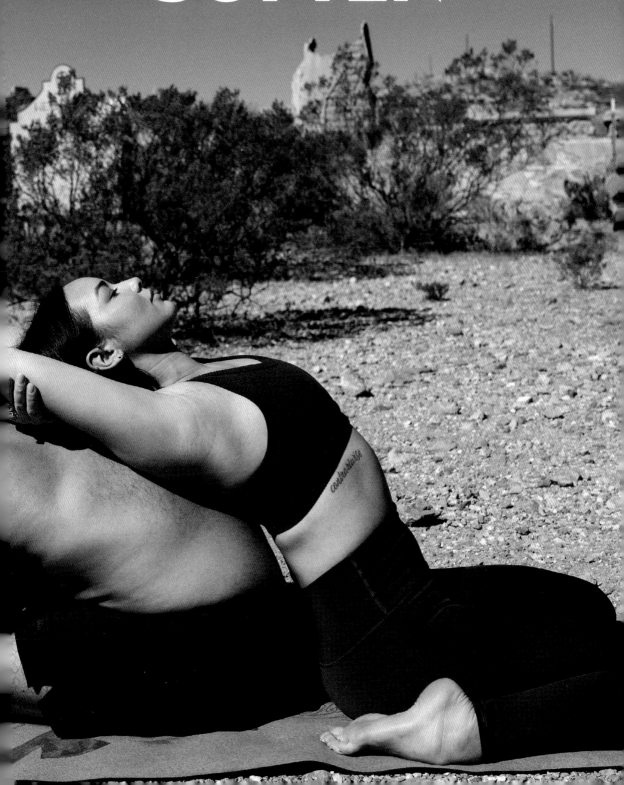

PART III
SOFTEN

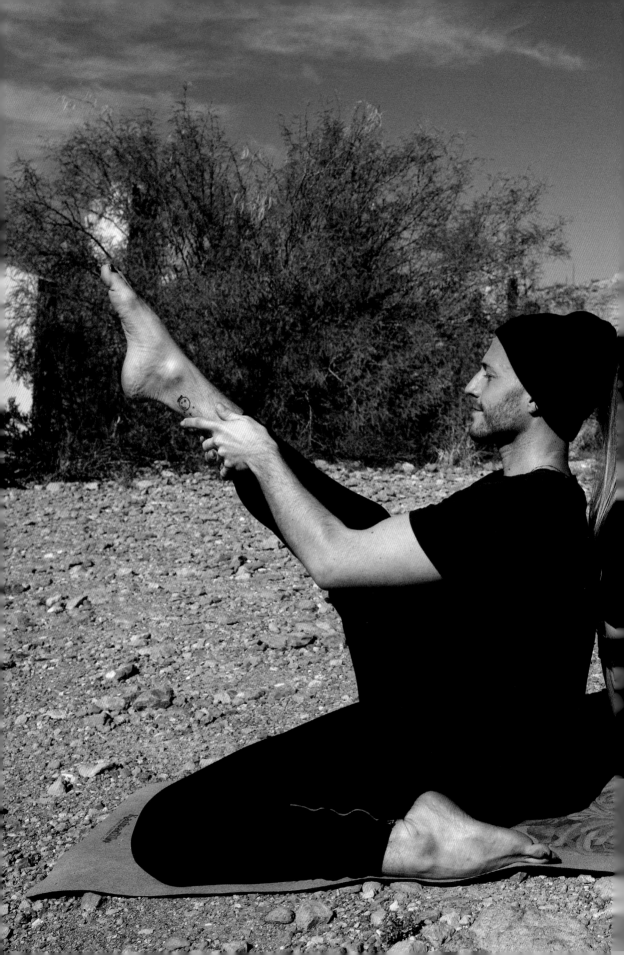

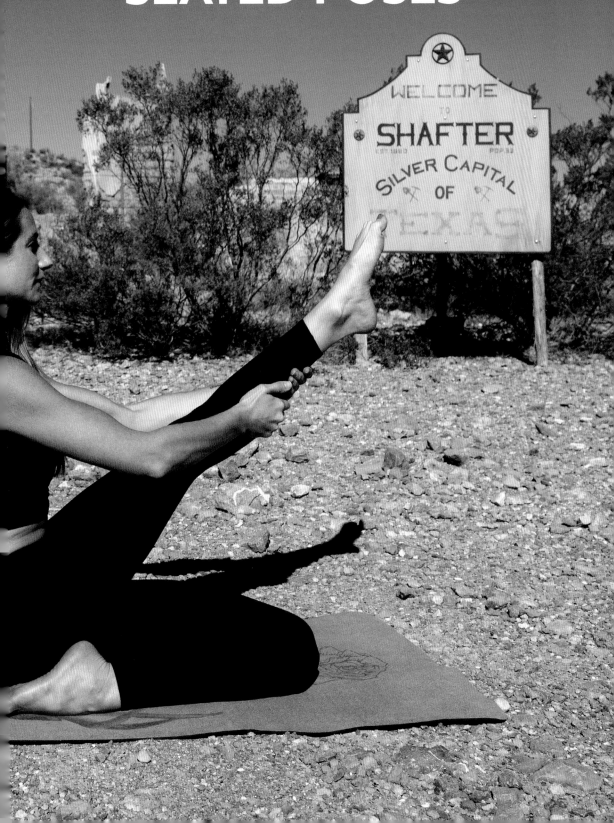

6
SEATED POSES

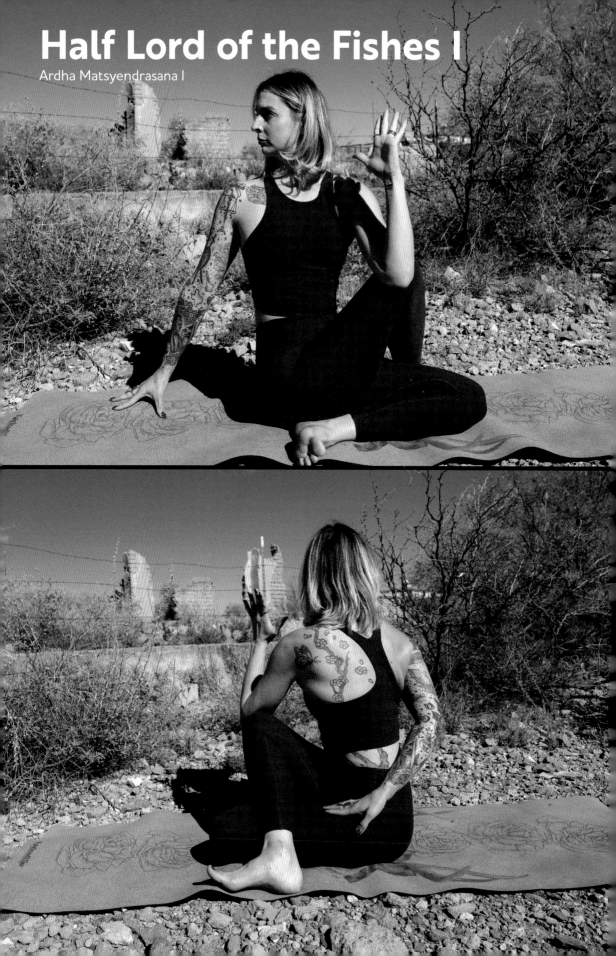

Half Lord of the Fishes I
Ardha Matsyendrasana I

About This Pose

This seated pose deeply stretches the outer hip of the bent leg while activating the inner thighs and many layers of muscles in the spine to create the twist. It is a great opportunity to breathe into the side of the rib cage as well as the back of the rib cage.

How To

- While seated with your legs stretched out in front of you, bring your right knee to your chest and place your right foot on the outside of your left thigh. Bend the left knee and pull the left foot in near your right hip. Squeeze your inner thighs together. Your sternum, pubic bone, and knees are more or less in line with one another.
- Place your right hand behind you and extend your left arm overhead. Inhale to lengthen the spine and left arm.
- Exhale and rotate your left ribs over your right thigh, hooking your upper left arm on the outside of the right thigh, keeping your palm open and fingers spread as if doing a "high five" with the left hand.
- Stay here and breathe as you hug the legs to the midline. Exhale and use your core muscles to deepen the twist. Relax the right hip toward the floor to lengthen the outside of your thigh and stretch the glutes.
- Internally rotate the upper right arm as you reach behind your back to place your finger pads on the top of your left thigh.

Variation

Half Lord of the Fishes With Extended Leg

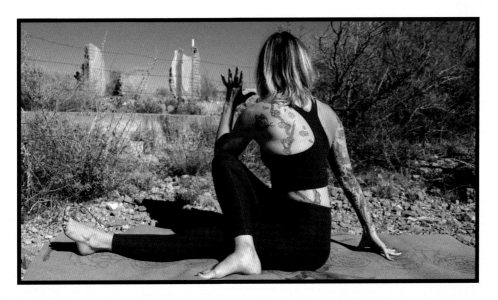

Follow the instructions for half lord of the fishes I, but instead of bending your left knee to place your left foot next to your right hip, keep your left leg long and extended on the floor in front of you.

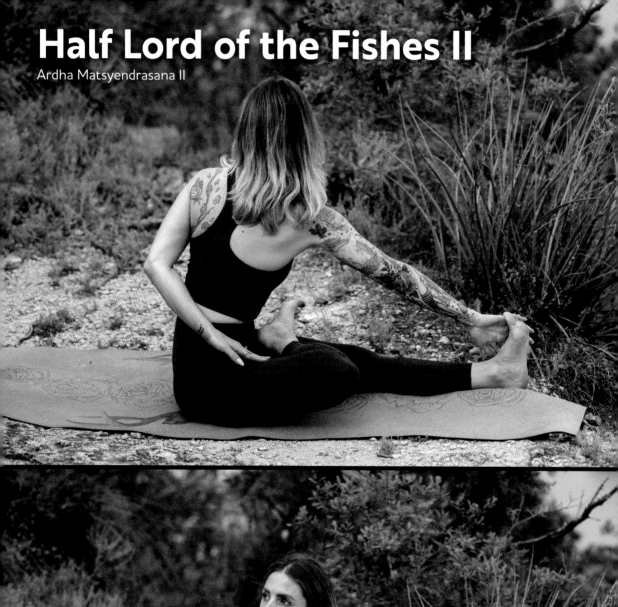

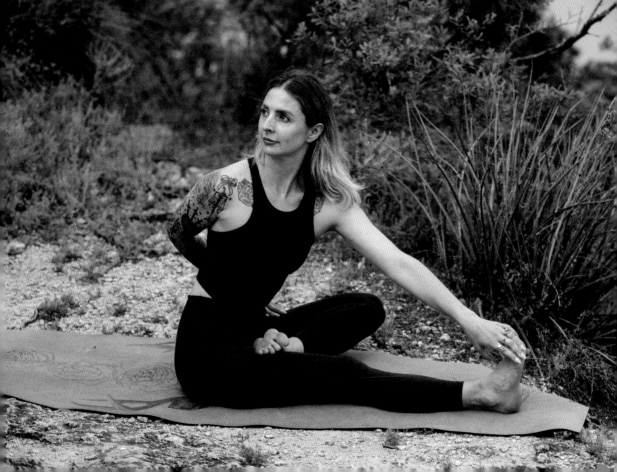

About This Pose

This variation incorporates a deep spinal twist, a lotus leg, a straight leg, and more of a forward bend. As such, this variation offers more stretch for the hamstrings and less stretch for the glutes, while still strengthening the muscles along the spine and the obliques. Be careful with your knees when practicing any poses with a lotus leg. The knees tend to make up for any lack of mobility in the hips, so ensure you are adequately warmed up and never rush the entrance into the pose.

How To

- While seated with your legs stretched out in front of you, bring your right knee to your chest and place your right foot on the floor alongside the inner left thigh. Holding your right shin with both hands, allow your knee to fall out to the side. Slide your knee farther to the side before gently lifting the right ankle to rest on your left hip crease. Engage your left quadricep and flex the toes of your left foot toward your face.
- As you inhale, lengthen the spine and sit up tall.
- As you exhale, twist your rib cage to the left and hinge forward to catch your outer left foot with your right hand.
- Internally rotate your left upper arm as you reach behind your back and clasp your right upper thigh.
- Stay here and breathe as you slowly deepen the twist. Activate the deep muscles of the lateral hip to keep the right knee down.
- Gaze over your left shoulder.

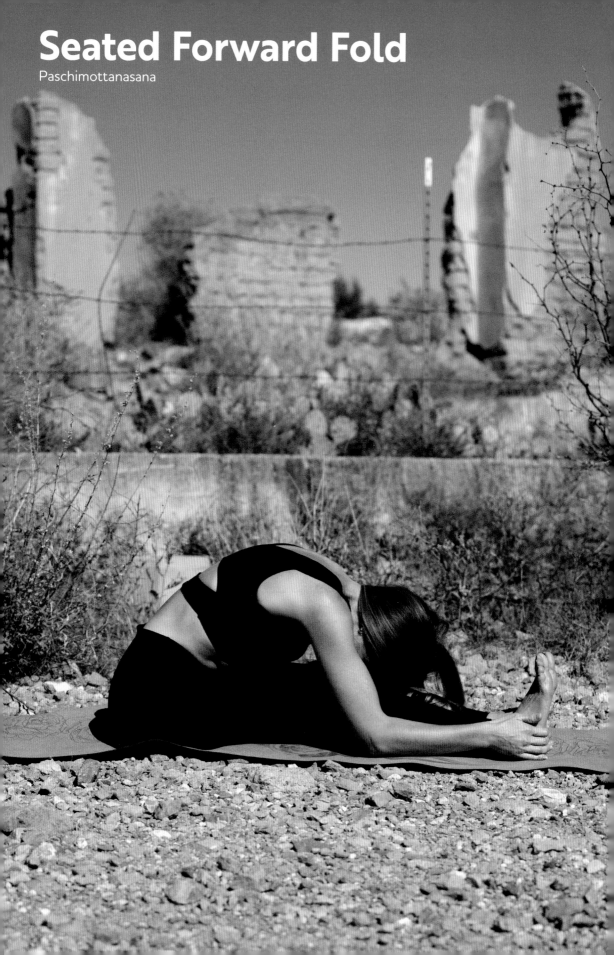

Seated Forward Fold
Paschimottanasana

About This Pose

This seated pose is a deep stretch for the entire posterior chain. You can build strength in the front of your body, particularly in the core and hip flexors. The symmetry of your legs means the pose is generally safer for those with sacroiliac joint issues, yet it can also feel more intense than asymmetrical poses such as janu sirsasana (head-to-knee forward bend).

How To

- Sit with your legs stretched out in front of you and your feet about hip-distance apart. Engage your quadriceps and pull your toes toward your nose.
- Inhale and lengthen your rib cage away from your hips without flaring the ribs out.
- Exhale as you hinge forward from your hips. Keep as much length in the spine as possible.
- Grab hold of your toes with your index and middle fingers, reach out to the heels or shins, or use a strap as a lasso around your feet.
- Gaze at your toes or relax your neck and close your eyes.

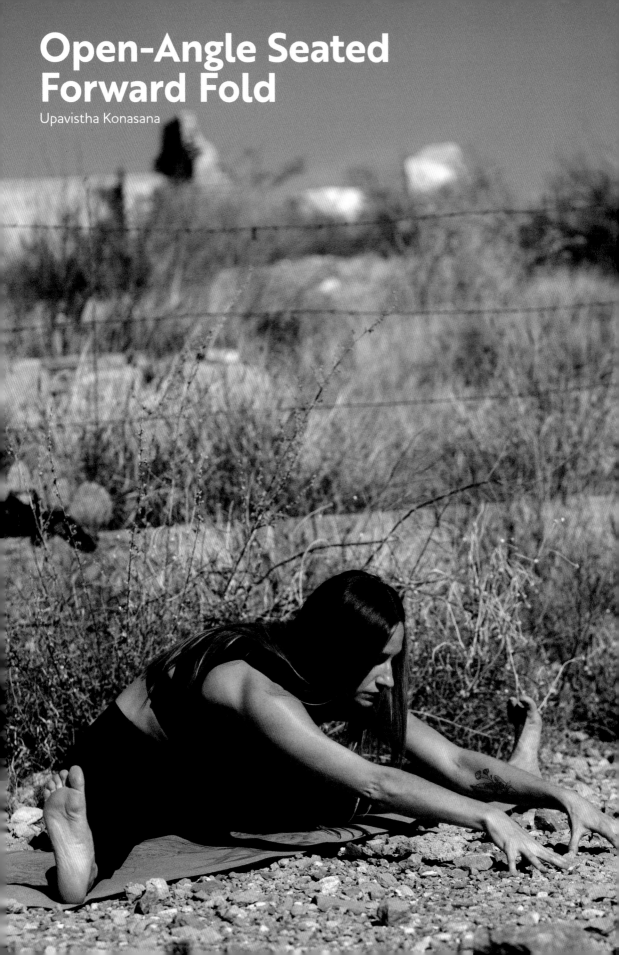

Open-Angle Seated Forward Fold

Upavistha Konasana

About This Pose

This seated forward bend, also known as straddle, is an accessible hamstring and inner thigh stretch and will strengthen the deep core and hip flexors. It is also an excellent preparation for advanced handstand entrances.

How To

- Sit with your legs stretched out in front of you, then open your legs out to the sides as far as your inner thighs can comfortably stretch. Point your toes or flex them toward your nose, whichever allows you to strongly engage the legs.
- With your hands on your legs, inhale and stretch your rib cage away from the pelvis.
- Exhale, engage the deep core, and hinge forward from the hips. Keep your spine long as you aim your chest toward the floor between your feet. You have the option to place your hands on the floor for support.
- Externally rotate your hips to activate the lateral hips and use the core and hip flexors to deepen your fold.

Variations

Open-Angle Seated Forward Fold With a Twist

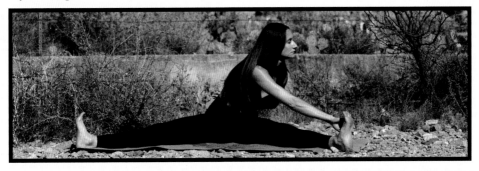

Feel free to play with adding a side bend or spinal twist, aiming to keep the hips evenly anchored throughout.

Open-Angle Seated Forward Fold With Lateral Flexion

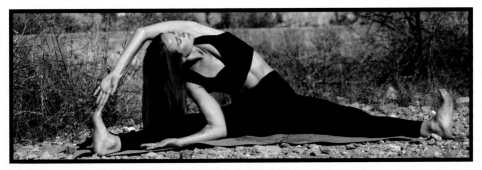

From open-angle seated forward fold, place a forearm against the inside of the same-side leg. Lean toward that side, finding lateral flexion in the spine, and lift the opposite arm overhead. Reach with the top hand toward the opposite foot while keeping the chest centered and squared forward. Maintain activation in both quadriceps and energize the feet as if they are pressing into a wall.

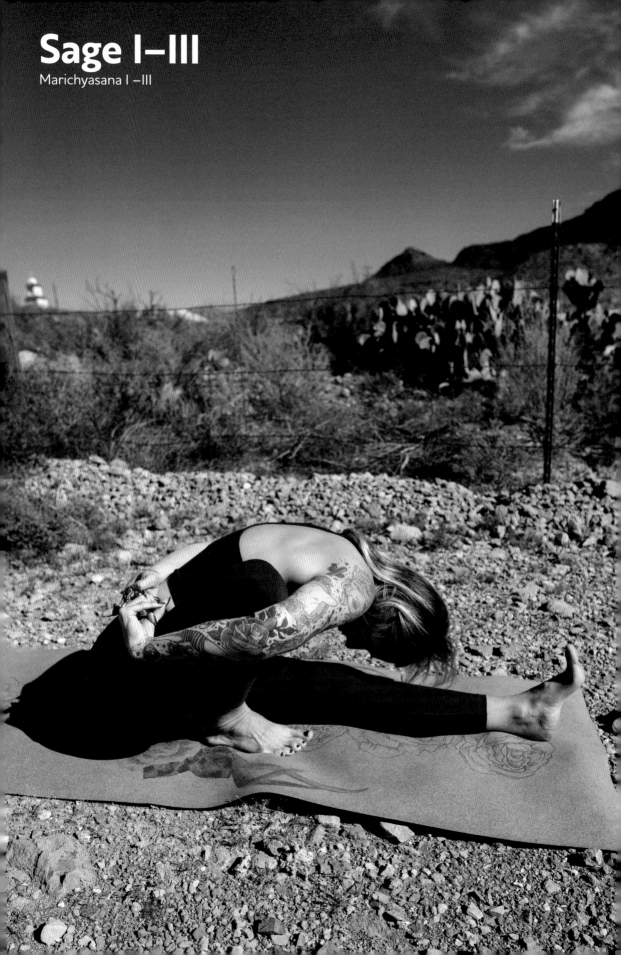

Sage I–III

Marichyasana I –III

About This Pose

This series of seated poses shares an asymmetry in the legs, deep forward bend, and bound arms. One of these poses (marichyasana II) includes a lotus-leg position in one leg, which is challenging all on its own—and now we add the arm bind. Although these poses show up in the primary series of ashtanga, they are by no means beginner level. The sage poses require strength in the rotator cuff, shoulders, and core while stretching the back extensors and hamstrings. A strap is extremely beneficial for the arm bind, and elevating your pelvis on a blanket can assist your lower-body positioning.

How To: Marichyasana I

- While seated with your legs stretched out in front of you, bring your right knee to your chest and place your right foot near the left inner thigh.
- Inhale to lengthen the spine and engage your left leg muscles.
- Exhale and hinge forward over your left leg, allowing the right knee to dip to the side enough that your torso can pass by.
- Extend your right arm forward, then internally rotate the bicep down as you reach the arm around and behind your right leg. Aim to get your shin to rest in your armpit.
- Either grab your left big toe with your left index and middle finger or internally rotate the left arm and reach back to clasp your right hand. Never force the bind because this action imposes a high demand on your shoulder mobility.
- Squeeze your right inner thigh in to your torso and relax your right hip toward the floor.
- Press your arm into your right shin as you lengthen your spine and relax your neck.

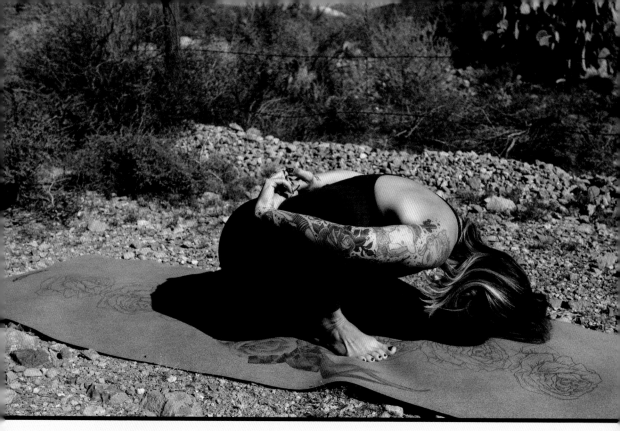

Variations

Marichyasana II

Follow the instructions for sage I, but instead of keeping your left leg extended on the floor, place your left foot into the crease at the front of your right thigh (at the hip flexor) to find lotus in the left leg. When you hinge forward, your chin is reaching toward your left bent knee.

Marichyasana III

- While seated with your legs stretched out in front of you, bring your right knee to your chest and place your foot near the left inner thigh. Firm up your left leg and activate your right inner thigh to keep the leg close to the midline.
- Place your right hand behind you and extend your left arm in the air. Inhale to lengthen the spine and left arm.
- Exhale and rotate your left ribs over your right thigh, hooking your upper left arm on the outside of the right leg.
- Stay here and breathe as you hug the legs to the midline. Exhale and use your core muscles to deepen the twist. Keep your sitz bones pressing down to anchor your hips into the mat.
- If that is going well, lean your upper body more to the right past your thigh as you internally rotate the left arm around your bent leg. Reach the back of your hand to your left hip. Actively press your left upper arm against your leg and rotate the rib cage.
- Internally rotate the right arm and reach behind your back to clasp your left hand. Never force the bind because doing so places a high demand on your shoulder mobility.
- Continue to activate the twist with the deep core and obliques rather than relying on the arms as leverage.

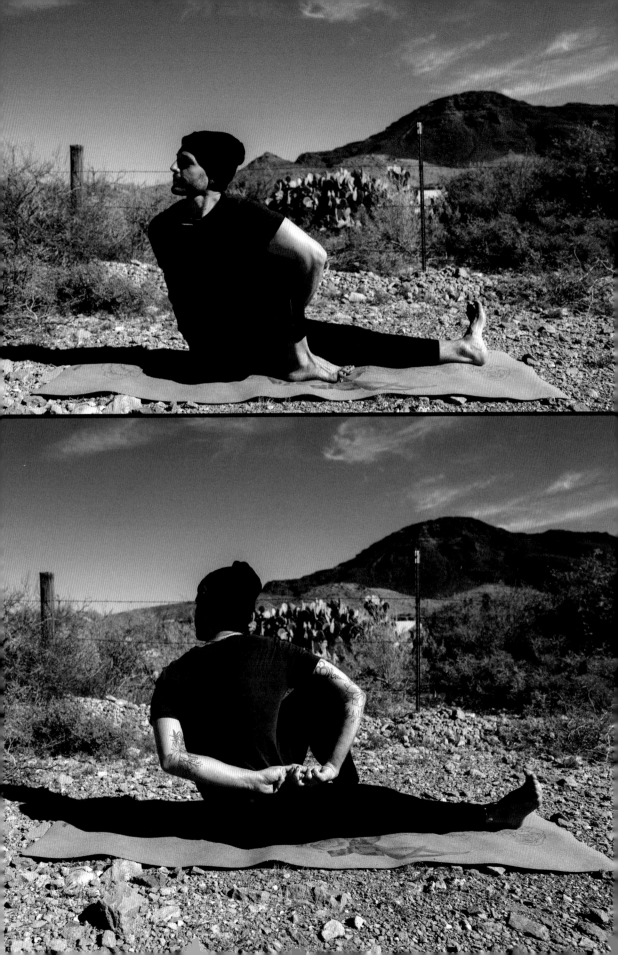

Front Splits
Hanumanasana

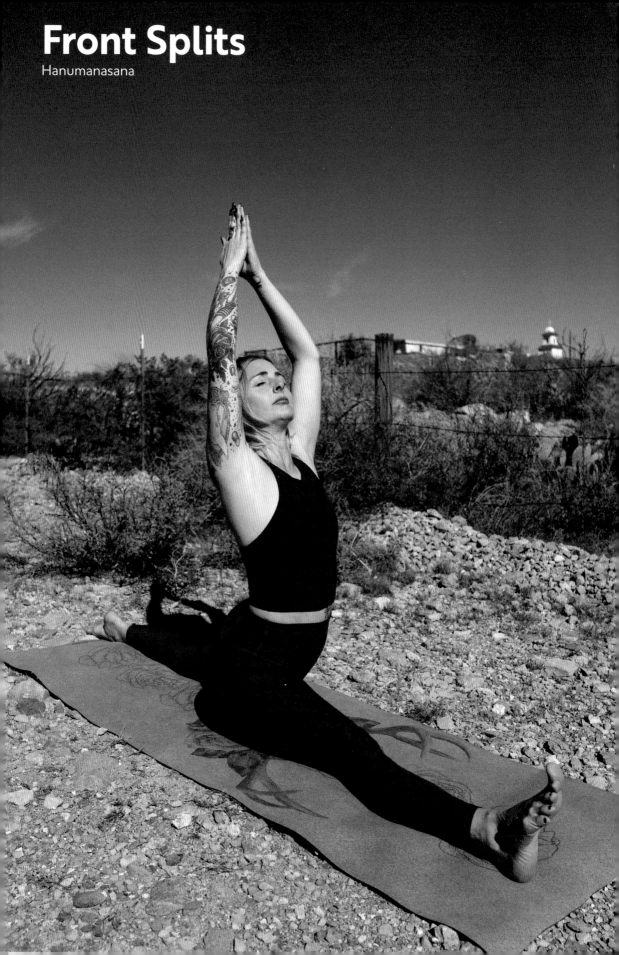

About This Pose

This is a wonderful pose to experience how to strengthen the opposing muscles to deepen the intended stretch. The hip flexors and quadriceps of the front leg contract to stretch the back of the leg, while the activation of the glutes of the back leg moves the hip into more extension to stretch the front side. Use your core to stabilize the pelvis and keep your spine lifted. Flexibility is one major factor; however, hip structure varies widely and will affect your pose.

How To

- From crescent low lunge, place your hands on the floor or on blocks beside your hips for stability. Tuck your back toes, lift the back knee, and inch your back leg farther back.
- Move your front foot farther forward a few inches at a time. Flex the top of your foot and toes toward your nose so you balance on the heel.
- With shoulders aligned over your hips and hands on the floor, engage the deep core and lift the front of your pelvis.
- Inhale and lengthen the rib cage up away from your hips. Press the front heel down to activate the hamstrings and isometrically pull the legs toward one another.
- Exhale from your deep core and press the legs in opposite directions, squeezing the quadriceps of your front leg and glutes of the back leg.
- Gaze forward and keep your neck long.
- Once your balance is steady, reach your arms overhead and encourage more lift of the rib cage.

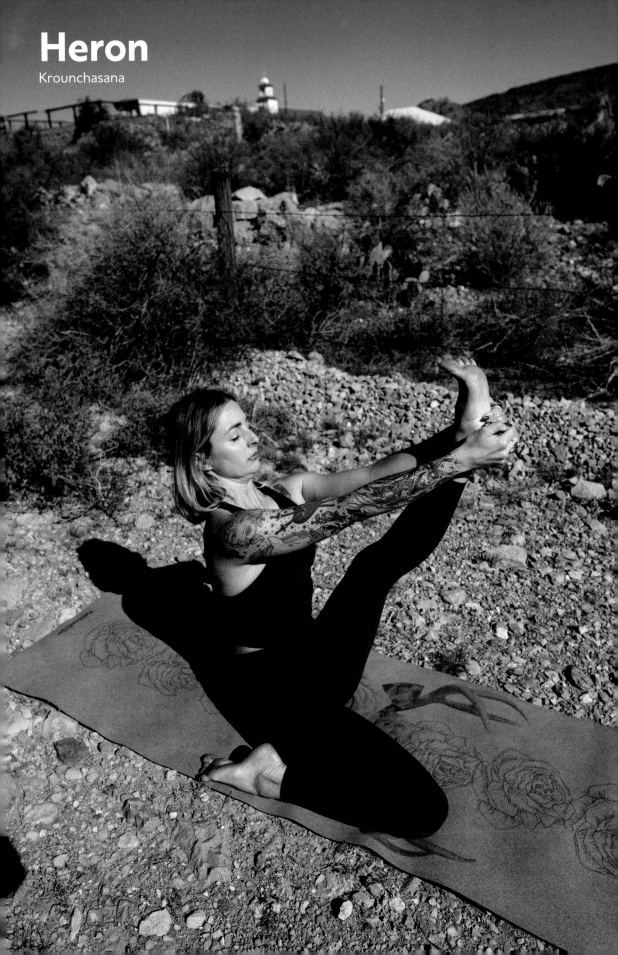

Heron
Krounchasana

About This Pose

Heron pose is a unique seated hamstring and hip stretch. Rather than lowering the upper body toward the leg and the floor using gravity for assistance, lift the leg and work to maintain an upright spine. That small change has an intense effect on the pose. Also, given that the opposite leg is anchored in hero pose—a quad stretch with hip internal rotation—the pelvis and lumbar spine will seem limited in their range of motion and you may experience different sensations in the lifted leg. This pose can also be done with a strap to help with balance while sitting upright and to increase flexibility in the extended leg's hamstring (see variation photo).

How To

- Sit with both legs stretched out in front of you. Bend the right knee and swing your right foot back to rest next to your hip like in hero pose, with the top of the foot on the mat and toes pointed behind you.
- Inhale to sit tall and press your hips into the floor.
- As you exhale, engage the deep core and use the hip flexors to hug your left knee to your chest so that you can grab your left foot from the sides with both hands.
- Squeeze your quadriceps and kick your left foot into your hand to extend the left leg upward.
- Actively bring your torso toward your left leg while simultaneously hugging the leg closer to your chest.
- Keep your spine long as your look up past your foot.

Variation

Heron With a Strap

If grabbing the foot of the extended leg is too much for your hamstrings, consider using a strap to bind around the foot of your lifted leg. As you squeeze your quadriceps and extend your leg upward, bring your hands on the strap as close to your lifted foot as possible, without rounding your back. Continue to engage your core to find balance.

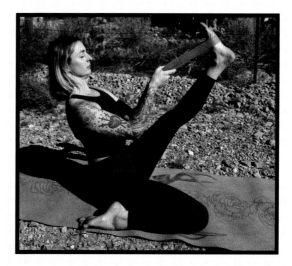

Three-Limb Intense Stretch

Triang Mukhaikapada Paschimottanasana

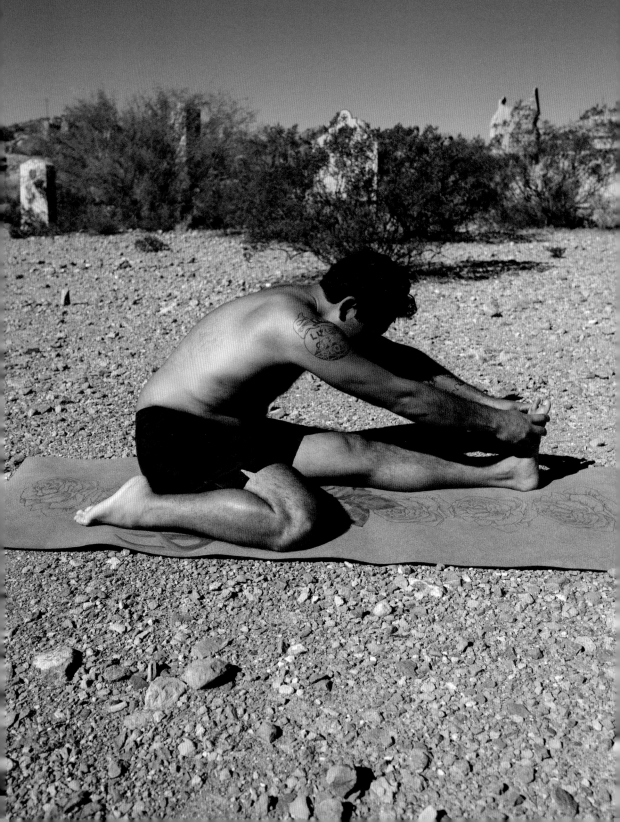

About This Pose

This pose incorporates three other poses—dandasana, virasana, and paschimotta-nasana—and is similar to heron in most of the shape, but owing to the change in orientation to gravity, the sensations can feel noticeably different. Like the name implies, this pose is an intense seated forward fold—not only because it deeply stretches the back of the leg and hips but also because it can feel awkward and unbalanced given the asymmetry of the lower body. The strong psoas contraction for deep hip flexion starts the journey to level out the hips. If you have access to a block or firm pillow (especially if you have any knee or ankle pain), prop your pelvis up to settle both hips equally. Although gravity assists in the folding action, working actively in this pose will strengthen the deep core and hip flexors.

How To

- Sit on the floor with your legs stretched out in front of you. Bend one knee and swing your foot back to rest next to your hip like in hero pose, with the top of the foot on the mat and the toes pointed behind you.
- Inhale to sit tall and press your hips into the floor.
- As you exhale, engage the deep core and bend forward at your hips, reaching both hands for your front foot.
- Squeeze the quadriceps of your straight leg and actively pull both thighs toward your chest using the core and hip flexors, especially the thigh of the bent leg to help anchor the inner hip to the ground.
- Gaze forward to your foot or down at your shin.

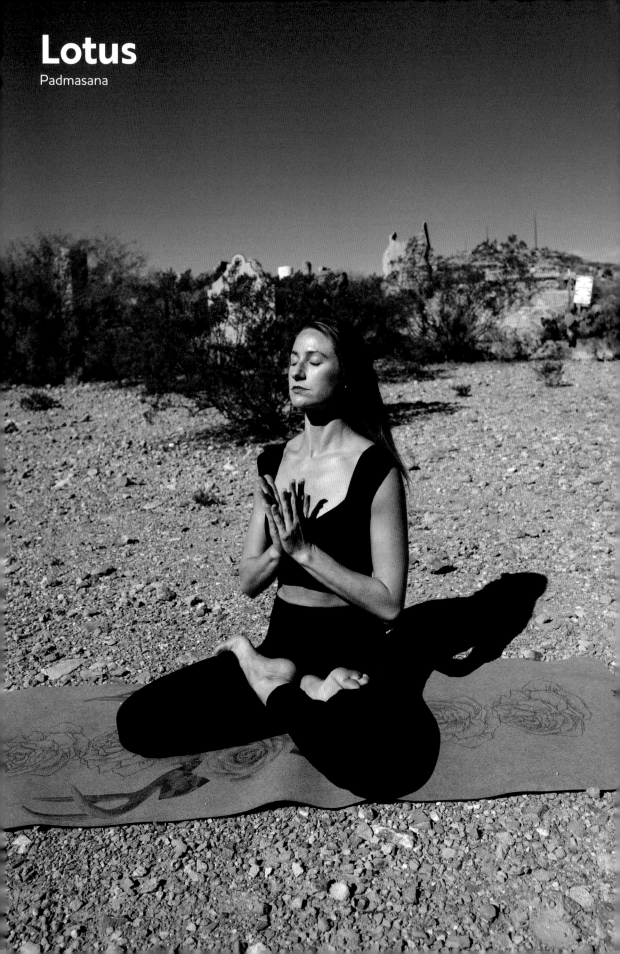

Lotus
Padmasana

About This Pose

Lotus requires both legs to externally rotate in the hip socket. The range of circular rotation of the femur in the hip joint will vary from person to person. The leg position is a result of a high degree of hip external rotation, and there is minimal torque on the knee (no more rotation than a few degrees).

How To

- Sit on the floor with your legs stretched out in front of you. Hug one knee into your chest and use your hands to squeeze the ankle tight against your hip.
- With the knee in this deep flexion, allow the hip to externally rotate and the knee to drop down toward the floor. Use your hands to guide your knee farther out to the side before lifting your foot to place it on the inner thigh of your opposite leg.
- Once in this position, slide your second foot in toward your lotus leg as you bend that knee out to the side. Once again with deep knee flexion, use your hands to guide your knee farther out to the side before lifting the ankle to slide it over the shin to rest on your opposite inner thigh.
- Push down with the outer edges of your feet into your inner thighs and activate the outer hips to move your knees closer to the floor.
- Gaze forward or down at your shins—or close your eyes.
- Your hands can rest on your lap or be held palm to palm in front of the heart.

Variation

Lotus Full Bind

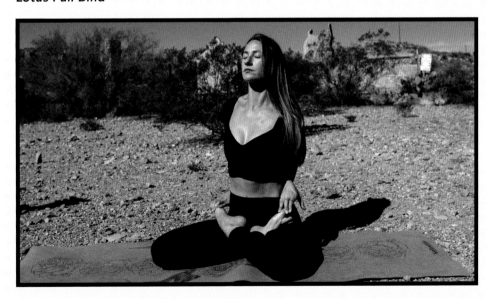

Once in lotus, wrap one arm behind your lower back as you internally rotate your bicep and grab the foot of the same side. Do the same with your other arm so that both arms are crossed behind your lower back. Grab the foot of the same side with your second hand. Continue to engage your core to sit erect.

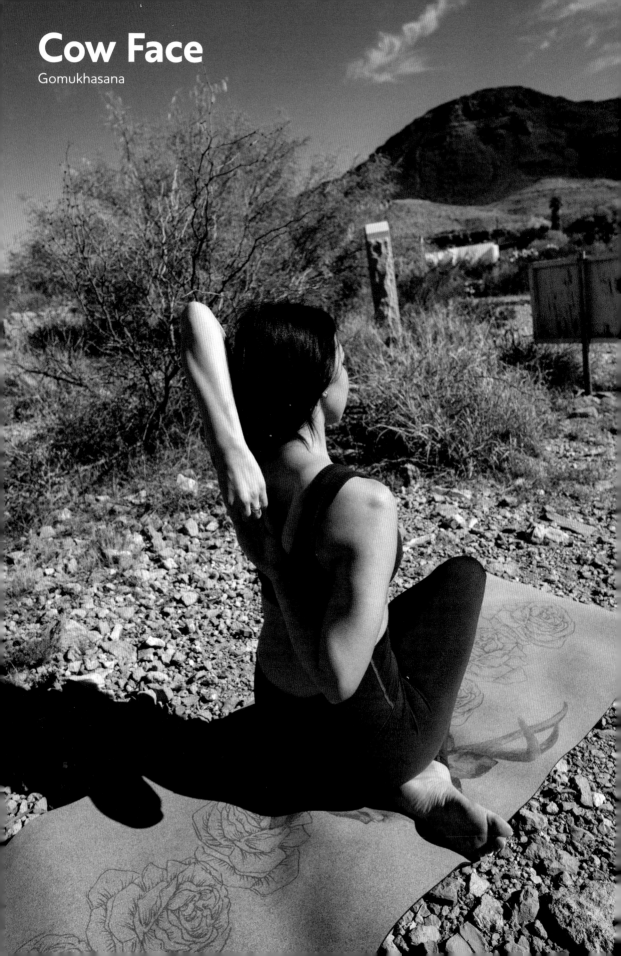

Cow Face
Gomukhasana

About This Pose

Cow face pose deeply stretches both the upper and lower body. The narrow angle of the thigh bones translates to a more concentrated stretch on the gluteus maximus and piriformis compared with wide-knee hip stretches. If you have knee issues, bring the feet closer to your hips to lessen the potential for twisting at the knee joint. You can also elevate your hips on a block or pillow. Healthy internal and external rotation is needed for the full arm bind, so use a strap between your hands as you build up your practice of this pose.

How To

- With both legs stretched out in front of you, cross your right shin over your left shin. Bend your knees to move your feet toward your hips.
- Slide your right knee over your left knee, going only so far as allows you to keep both sitz bones anchored to the floor and have zero pinching or similar sensation in your knees.
- Sit up tall and reach your arms out to the sides like the letter "T."
- Internally rotate your right arm and place the back of your right hand on your mid to lower back, with the fingers pointing up.
- Externally rotate your left arm as your reach overhead and bend your elbow so your left palm connects to your upper back. Eventually clasp your fingers together but do not force the bind; even without it, enjoy the deep stretch in your arms and shoulders.
- Inhale and expand your back ribs and slightly lift your back ribs up from the low back so that you maintain a neutral spine.
- Exhale and engage the deep core and pelvic floor to stabilize your pelvis and keep the spine lifted.

Head-to-Knee Forward Bend

Janu Sirsasana

About This Pose

As the name implies, this is a seated pose in which you bend forward to touch your head to your knee or beyond, depending on your flexibility and the length of your spine and legs. It also incorporates a spinal twist as you rotate over your extended leg for a deep stretch in the opposite-side lower back and hip. The arms-overhead position allows for deep expansion in the rib cage with every inhale. In addition to using gravity to assist the fold, actively contract the muscles in your core and hip flexors to deepen the stretch in the back and hamstrings.

How To

- Seated with your legs stretched out in front of you, bend the right leg and bring your right foot in to rest against your upper left inner thigh, allowing your right knee to drop out to the side. Engage the quadriceps of your extended left leg and flex the left foot to bring your toes toward your nose.
- Inhale and extend your arms overhead, gathering maximum length in your upper body.
- Exhale, engage the deep core, rotate your torso to face the straight leg, and hinge forward. Grab your shin or foot—wherever you can reach comfortably.
- Gaze at your shin or close your eyes.
- Inhale to lengthen the spine and expand your side ribs. Exhale to contract the lower core and hip flexors of your straight leg.

Plow

Halasana

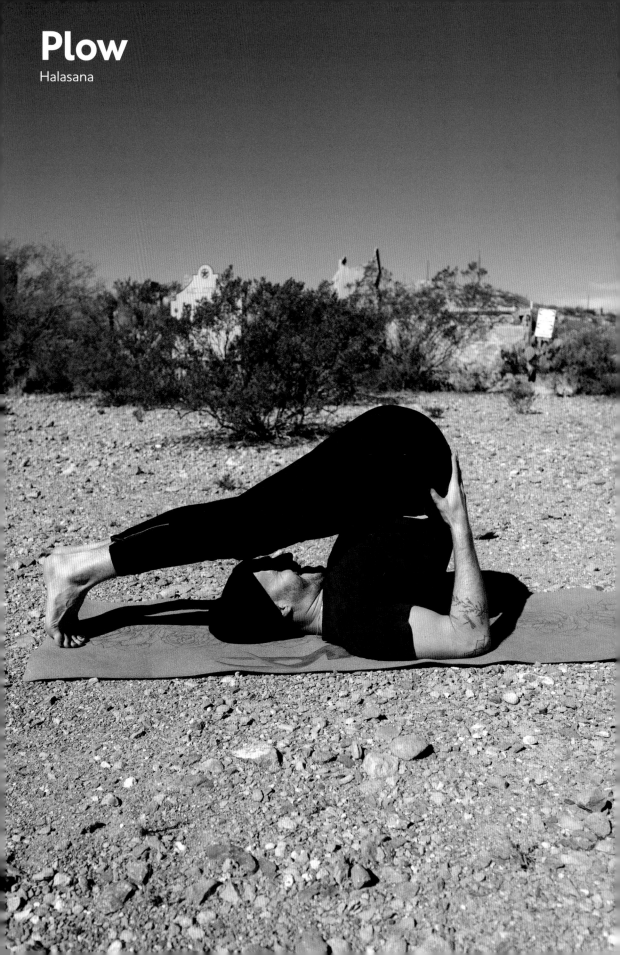

About This Pose

Plow is a deep stretch for the entire posterior chain. It strengthens shoulder extension and the deep core while allowing more space to breathe into the lower half of the rib cage. Like shoulder stand, this pose is best used only when you have blankets available—both out of caution for the cervical spine and for comfort, which in turn allows more time in the pose. From a functional standpoint, most people can flex easily at the C6-C7 and T1 vertebrae (the base of the neck) but not so easily in the middle thoracic to lumbar region. The props will lessen the emphasis on that portion of your neck and direct more of your effort toward the larger bones of the spine, which can yield more benefits.

How To

- Lie down on your back, with your arms next to your body and legs straight.
- On an exhale, engage the deep core, push your arms into the floor, and swing your legs up and over your head.
- Once your feet find the floor, engage the quadriceps to straighten your knees and bring your legs together—or no wider than parallel.
- Inhale and expand the back and sides of your rib cage. Exhale from the deep core. This may be a challenge because the front rib cage movement is limited by the shape of the pose.
- Your arms may remain straight with your hands down on the floor. Or, if it is comfortable for your shoulders, you can move your straight arms closer together to interlace your fingers behind your back. If you are interlacing your fingers, press down through the pinky finger edge of your hands and wrists.
- Gaze up at your legs and avoid rotating your head left or right.

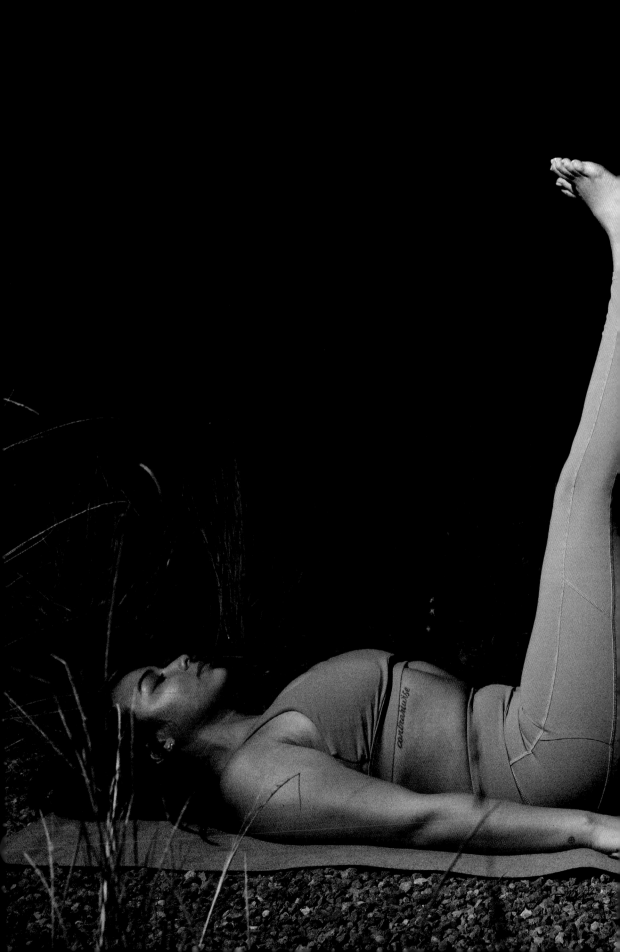

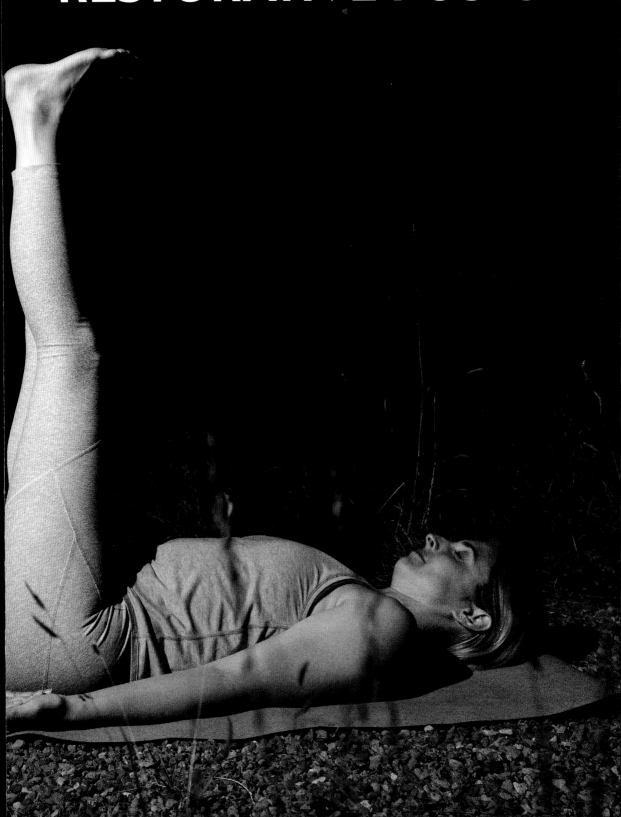

RESTORATIVE POSES

Supported Bridge
Salamba Setu Bandhasana

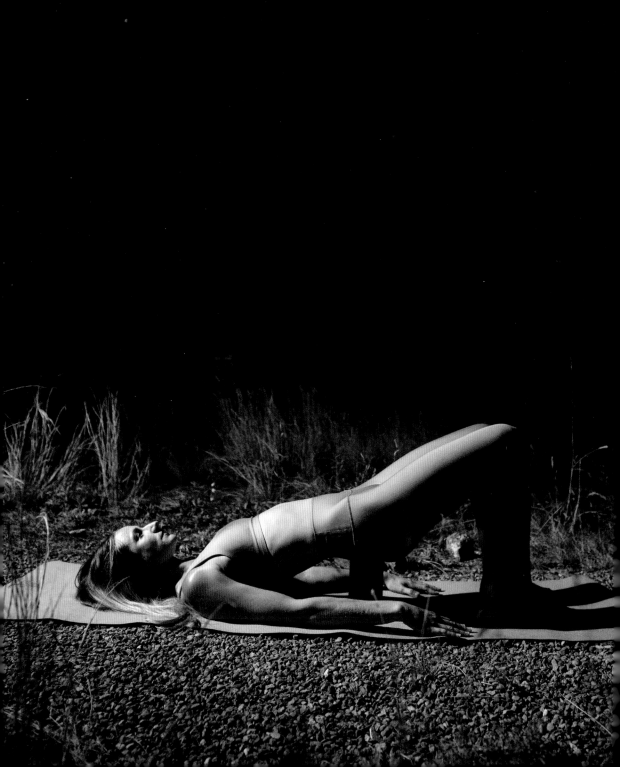

About This Pose

This version of bridge pose uses a prop, such as a block or firm bolster, to support the weight of your pelvis and allow you to gently stretch the chest, shoulders, abdominals, and front of the hips. With your hips above your head and the neck flexed, the nervous system is downregulated, which promotes relaxation.

How To

- Lying down on your back, bend your knees to place your feet on the floor about hip-distance apart.
- Push your feet down to lift your pelvis; place a block or firm bolster underneath. Ideally, the pelvis will be in a neutral position relative to the floor to avoid excessive strain in the lower back.
- The higher your prop, the more stretch you will feel in the front of the hips, thighs, and abdominals. This should be a fairly comfortable position you can stay in for several minutes.
- Wiggle your shoulders together behind your back to lift your chest toward your chin.
- Stay in position and breathe. When you are ready to come down, push through your feet to lift your hips; remove the block. Gently lower yourself down to the floor and rest.

Reclined Hero

Supta Virasana

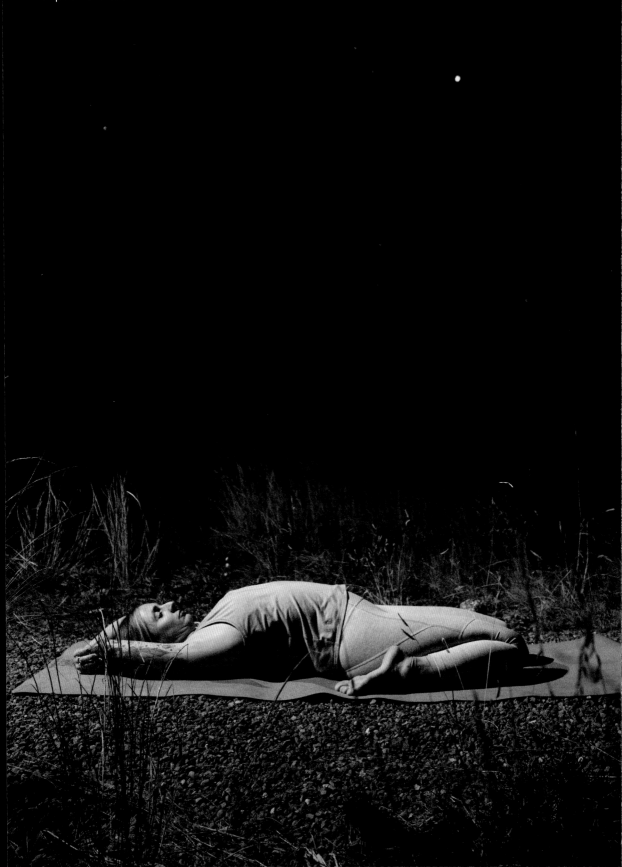

About This Pose

As the name suggests, this is a reclined version of the seated hero pose. Lying supine increases the stretch for the hip flexors and thighs, as well as adding a subtle backbend to the shape. While the full reclined variation can be quite intense, supporting your spine with a prop such as a bolster makes this pose sustainable for several minutes (see variation photo).

How To

- Sitting in hero pose, extend your arms behind you for support as you lean back and scoop the tailbone under. This adjustment alone might be enough sensation, so feel free to stay and breathe here.
- Drop down onto your elbows to recline farther. Engage the lower core and be mindful of any pinching sensation in your lower back.
- Slowly lower your shoulders and head to the ground.
- Inhale to lengthen the rib cage away from the pelvis. Exhale, draw the deep core in, and settle into the floor.
- The arms can rest by your sides or reach overhead to grab the opposite elbows. Inhale to encourage more expansion in the side ribs.
- Gaze up or close your eyes.

Variation

Reclined Hero With Props

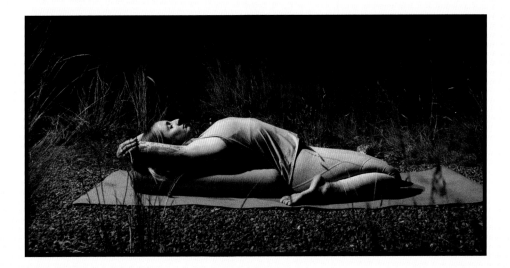

Sitting in hero pose, place a bolster behind your back with the short edge flush with your sacrum. As you lie back, your upper body will be supported by the bolster, decreasing the intensity on the quadriceps and psoas. Rest your arms by your sides or clasp the opposite elbows behind your head. Gaze up or close your eyes.

Reclined Big Toe A and B

Supta Padangusthasana A and B

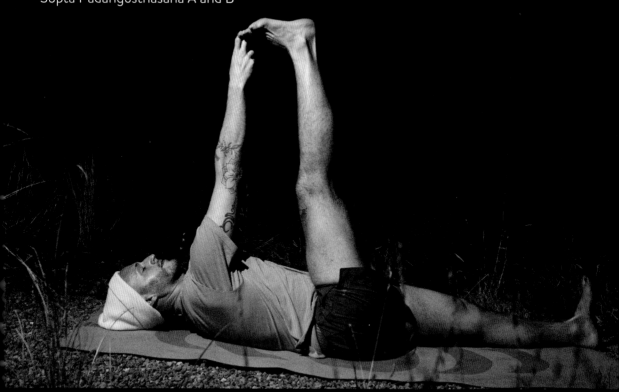

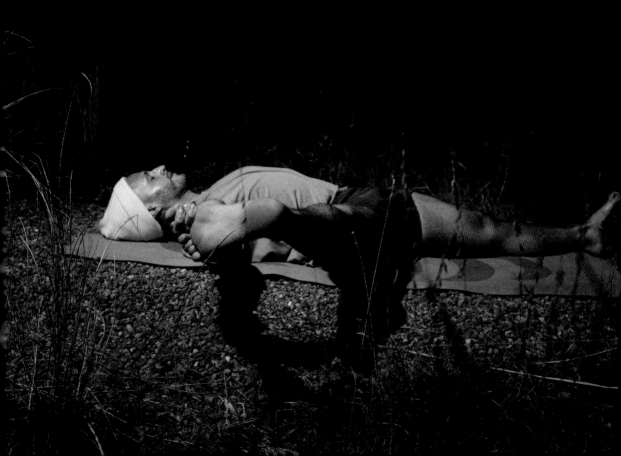

About This Pose

I prefer this reclined variation on big-toe pose over its standing counterpart, not because it requires less strength to balance (although that is a bonus), but because there is more of a sense of how the rest of your body is behaving in the pose since you can feel it on the ground. This usually means less depth because the hips and lower back are not compensating to find more range. It also allows for an opening of the hip flexor on the anchored leg. Even though you are reclined, this pose will strengthen the abdominals and hip flexors while stretching the hamstrings, calves, and feet. You can use a strap here so that the shoulders and head rest comfortably, with your knee straight. For reclined big toe B (see second photo), add a deep activation of the lateral hip to stretch the inner thigh as you extend your leg to the side.

How To

- Lie down on your back, with legs extended. Flex your left foot and stretch out through the back of the leg and heel.
- Exhale to engage the deep core as you bring your right knee to your chest. Grab hold of your big toe with the index finger, middle finger, and thumb.
- Kick your right heel upward and squeeze the quadriceps to straighten your knee.
- Relax your head and shoulders on the floor and gently loosen your grip on the big toe. Exhale to connect to the deep core and engage the hip flexors to maintain the height of your leg. Aim to bring your straight right leg closer to your face without changing your lower back or pelvis positions.
- Pull the top of your feet and toes toward your face to deepen the calf stretch.
- For reclined big toe B, anchor both hips and shoulders to the floor as you open your right leg out to the right. Kick out through both heels to lengthen the backs of your legs. Use the obliques to gently turn your torso in the opposite direction so hips and shoulders both remain in contact with the floor.

Revolved Reclined Big Toe

Parivrtta Supta Padangusthasana

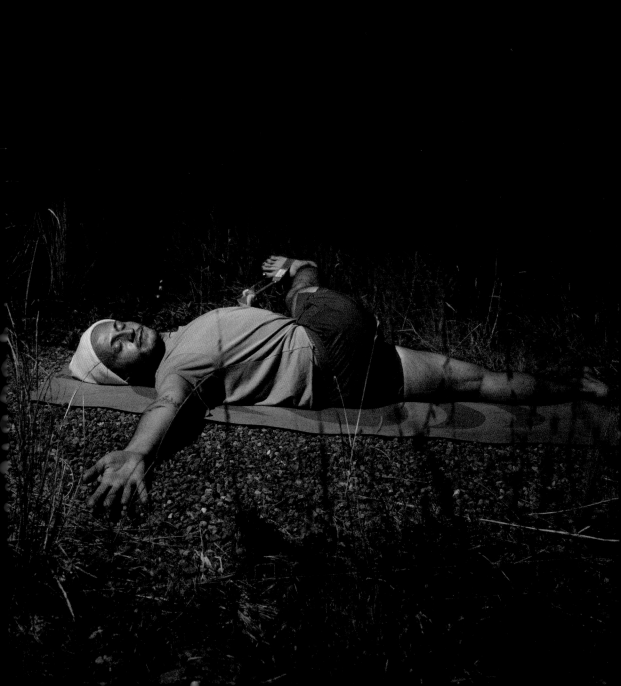

About This Pose

This twist variation on big-toe pose adds a stretch to the outer leg and hip while strengthening the obliques and deep spinal muscles. This is especially useful for runners and cyclists. Holding a strap around your foot makes the twist more accessible and generally allows you to be more comfortable and sustain the pose for a longer time. Considering how similar this pose is to revolved half moon, you could use this pose as a warm-up rather than a cool-down to focus on the spinal twist aspect before adding elements of balance and strength.

How To

- On the right side, from reclined big toe A, grab the big toe with your opposite hand or place your foot in a strap and grab the strap with both hands. Aim to relax your shoulders and head on the floor.
- After a few breaths, bring the leg across your body to the left, allowing your hips to align one hip bone over the other. If you are using a strap, it will be in your left hand as you let go with the right.
- Press out through both heels and draw your top hip bone down away from the bottom of your rib cage to lengthen the left side of your waist.
- Rotate your right ribs and shoulder back to the floor if they lifted up during the transition.
- Extend the right arm out to the right and rotate to look past your hand if it is comfortable on your neck.

Gentle Reclined Spinal Twist
Supta Matsyendrasana

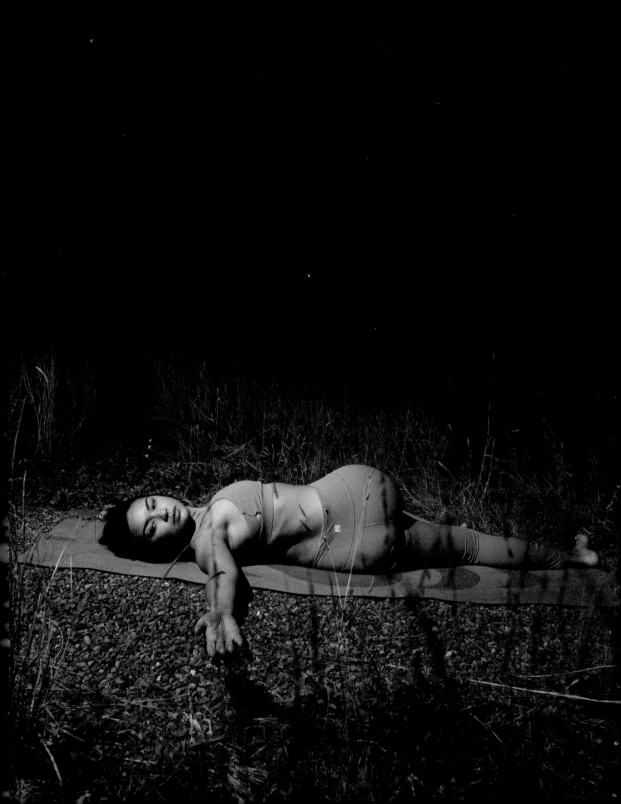

About This Pose

This twist is a more accessible—and perhaps more comfortable—version of revolved reclined big toe. Without the intensity of the hamstring stretch, you can focus on the spinal twist and stretching open the chest and the outer hip. Propping the twisted leg on a bolster or blocks can be helpful when holding this pose for an extended time.

How To

- Lie down on your back, with legs extended. Flex your left foot and stretch out through the back of the leg and heel.
- Exhale to engage the deep core as you bring your right knee to your chest. Grab hold of your knee or shin.
- Keep the shoulders on the floor as you use your left hand to swing your knee across to the left until your hips are aligned with one hip bone above the other. Your knee may or may not reach the floor. Never force it.
- Inhale to expand the rib cage and lengthen both sides of your torso. Encourage your top hip to move toward the foot of your mat and keep the hips aligned one on top of the other.
- Exhale and engage the core to deepen the twist. Turn your right rib cage and shoulder down toward the floor.
- Extend your right arm out to the right and gaze past your hand if that is comfortable for your neck.

Seated Baby Cradle

Hindolasana

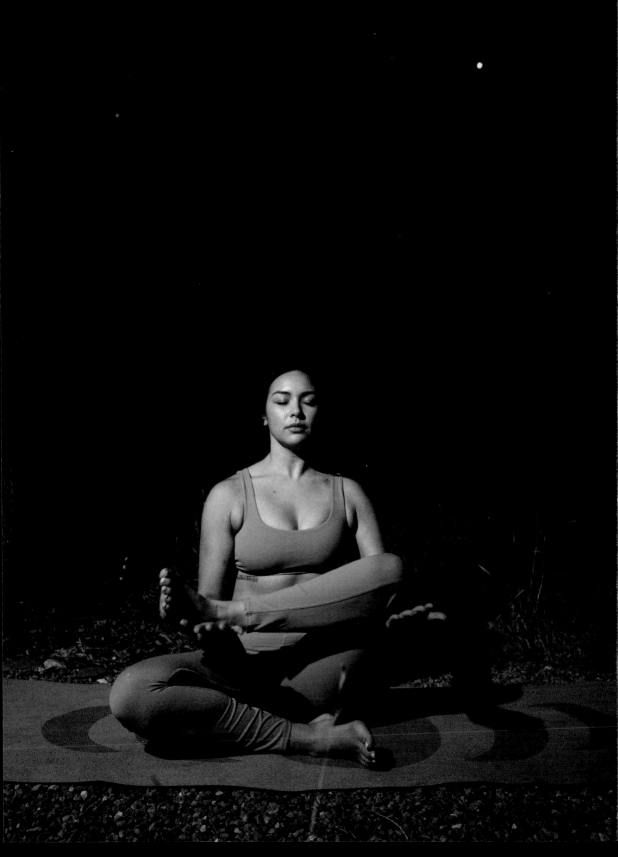

About This Pose

This seated pose deeply stretches the gluteus maximus and inner thighs while training the core to keep your spine upright. This pose is often used as an entrance to several arm balancing poses such as flying pigeon and eight-angle. Once you have reached the end of your range of motion in the hip, the knee will often twist or side bend as you attempt to deepen the pose. This could lead to major problems down the road. However, compared with seated hip stretches like one-legged king pigeon I, problems are *less* likely to happen, given that gravity is not tempting you to sink deeper into the pose. It can therefore be a useful substitute in your practice.

How To

- From a seated position, cradle your top leg with both arms. Your foot will nestle into the crook of your opposite elbow. Keep the toes and ankle flexed as you press the pinky-toe side of your foot into the elbow crease.

- The deep external rotation and flexion that allows the inner leg to touch the chest should come from the hip—*not* from the knee. Keep one hand under your foot and one hand under your knee, with your leg farther from your chest if you have knee issues. Stop before you feel any painful or uncomfortable sensation there or you cannot sit upright.

- Engage the deep core, sit up tall, and relax your shoulders as you gently rock your leg side to side.

Revolved Abdomen

Jathara Parivartanasana

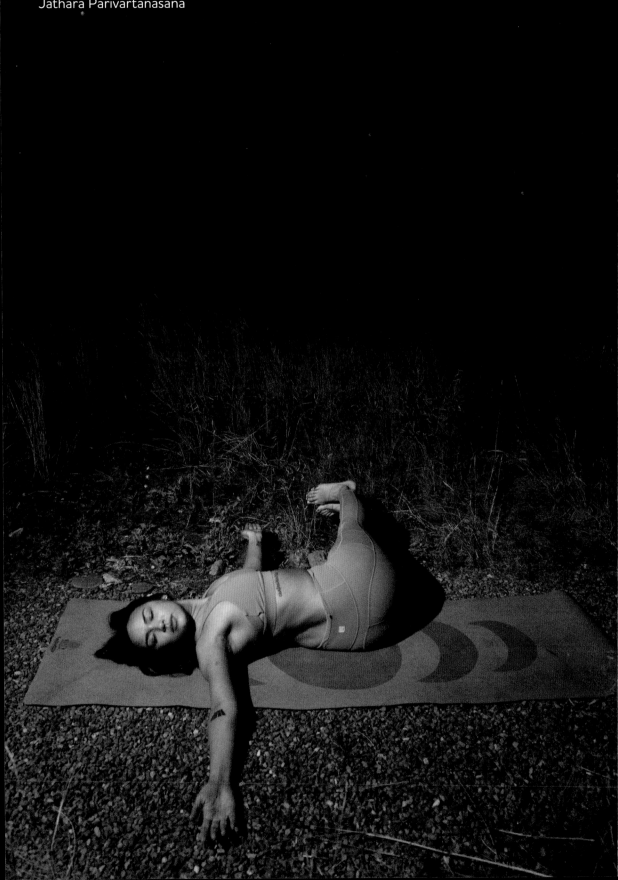

About This Pose

This pose offers different sensations because the legs are symmetrical rather than separated as in revolved reclined big toe. The action of squeezing the legs together and rotating the spine strengthens the adductors, obliques, and deep spinal rotators while the outer hips, latissimus, and chest are lengthened. Bending your knees is an excellent adjustment that can decrease the intensity for your hamstrings, lower back, and sacroiliac joints.

How To

- Lie down on your back with your knees bent and feet flat on the floor. Extend your arms out to create a "T" shape and turn the palms up or down.
- Exhale to engage the deep core and extend your flexed feet straight up in the air.
- Lower both legs to one side so that your hips, knees, and ankles are aligned top over bottom. If the top leg appears shorter, the hips are not vertical, so extend out more through the entire top leg and deepen the twist to align your top hip over your bottom hip and keep the legs together as if you have one leg.
- Stay in position for several breaths, inhaling to lengthen the rib cage away from the hips and exhaling to twist the opposite-side ribs and shoulder back toward the floor.
- Gaze up or past your opposite arm if it is comfortable for your neck.
- When you are ready to change sides, exhale to engage the core and use that core strength to swing your legs back to center. If you have any low back concerns, slide your top leg across the floor to the center of your mat; your hips will naturally follow to return to their original position.

Reclined Bound Angle

Supta Baddha Konasana

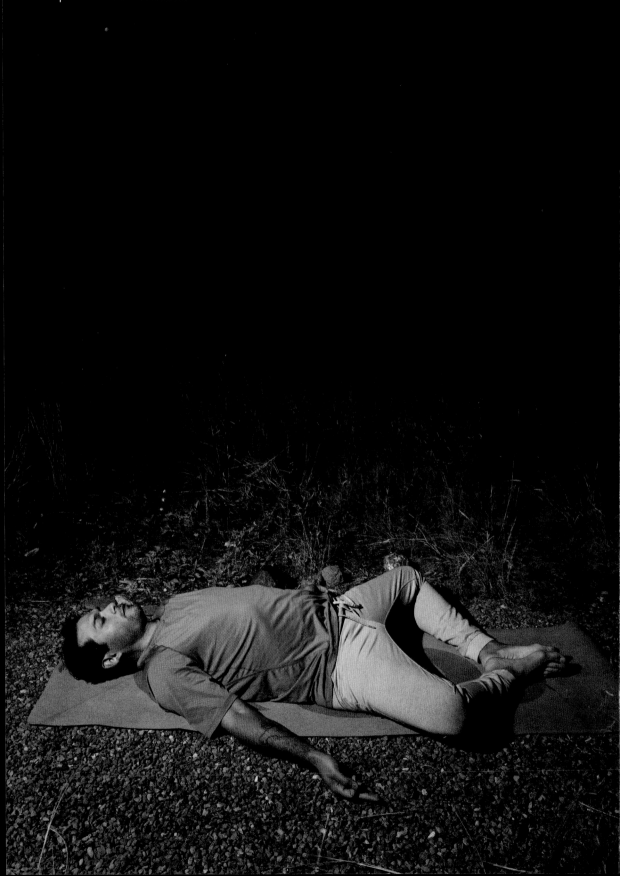

About This Pose

Although this pose is typically sequenced at the end of practice as a cool-down, it would also be useful as a gentle warm-up pose for the inner thigh lengthening needed for standing poses such as warrior II, side angle, and half moon. As a restorative pose, you can use a block under each knee or blankets under your spine to make the pose sustainable for longer periods of time.

How To

- Lie down on your back and place the soles of your feet on the floor. Take a breath or two here to find a neutral position for your spine and pelvis so there is no excessive arch in the lower back and the bottom ribs can relax toward the floor.
- Move the feet toward each other, allowing the knees to lower out to the sides so the soles of your feet can press together. Notice any changes in your pelvis position and adjust the placement of your feet as needed to find the neutral shape.
- Rest your arms by your sides, out like a "T," or overhead for varying stretches in the shoulders and chest.
- Inhale to lengthen the rib cage away from the hips.
- Exhale and relax the weight of your legs, hips, ribs, and head into the floor.

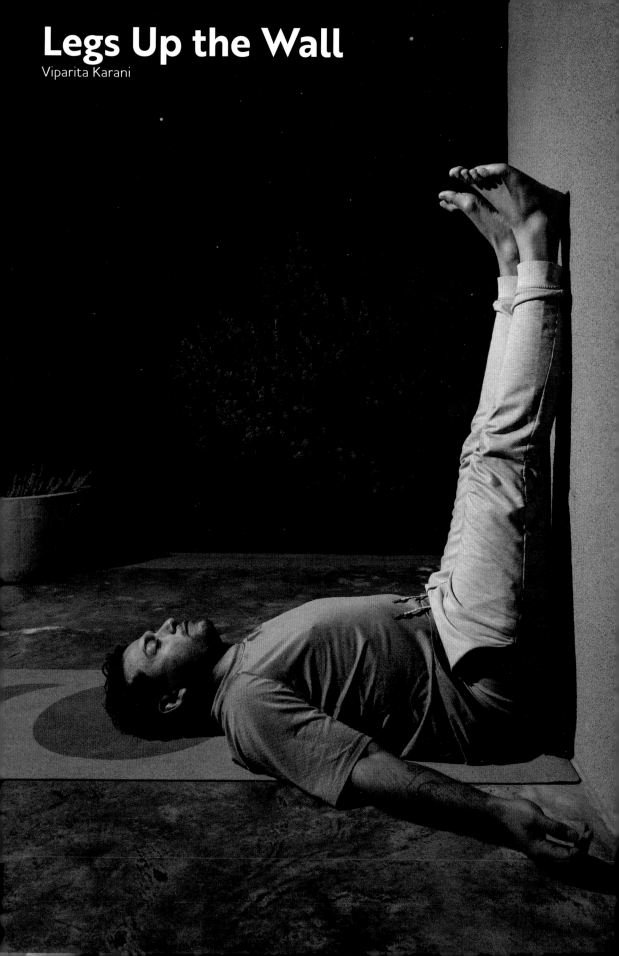

Legs Up the Wall
Viparita Karani

About This Pose

This pose is the perfect pose for any time of day. This pose helps with rebalancing the nervous system and promotes relaxation. However, you can use this pose when you need help feeling more energized, as this pose also promotes circulation. It's the best of both worlds! It is the most accessible inversion, so you can receive the benefits without any strain on your head, neck, or shoulders. This inversion greatly improves the circulation of bodily fluids and can ease lower back distress.

How To

- Sit on the floor parallel with a wall so one shoulder and hip are close to or touching the wall. Lower to the floor in a side-lying fetal position with your hips and feet near the wall and your knees curled in toward your chest.
- After a breath or two, shift onto your back and walk your feet up the wall until your legs are straight.
- Your pelvis, rib cage, and head are on the floor, with the legs together or hip-distance apart. Allow a comfortable slight bend in your knees. If the stretch on the back of your legs is too much or the hips cannot be on the ground, slide away from the wall a few inches.
- Spend a few minutes breathing and relaxing the weight of your entire body.

Constructive Rest
Savasana (Variation)

About This Pose

This pose is a newer addition to the collection of commonly practiced modern yoga poses that has been borrowed and integrated from the Alexander technique. It is a semi-supine position that can be more restful for the lower back and pelvis between poses, and it is a wonderful option if lying flat in savasana, or corpse pose, is uncomfortable or not accessible. With the feet on the floor and the hips in some flexion, the lower body is more grounded, and the lower back can lengthen without the pull from the hip flexors. In this position with the knees touching, you incorporate a subtle internal rotation at the hip joint, which is an excellent counterbalance to the numerous external rotation and backbend postures.

How To

- Sit on the floor, with your legs stretched out in front of you. Gently roll onto one side and bring your knees toward your chest. Rest in this side-lying position for a breath or two.
- Roll onto your back and settle your head on the floor or a pillow, with the feet on the floor hip-distance apart and the knees pointing up.
- Bring your knees to touch each other; move your feet to a narrower spread if this changes your pelvis position.
- With every exhale, allow your weight to settle more into the floor, relaxing the deep muscles of the pelvis so the lower back can decompress.
- Stay here as long as you like and are comfortable, allowing for a deeper sense of relaxation over time.

Corpse
Savasana

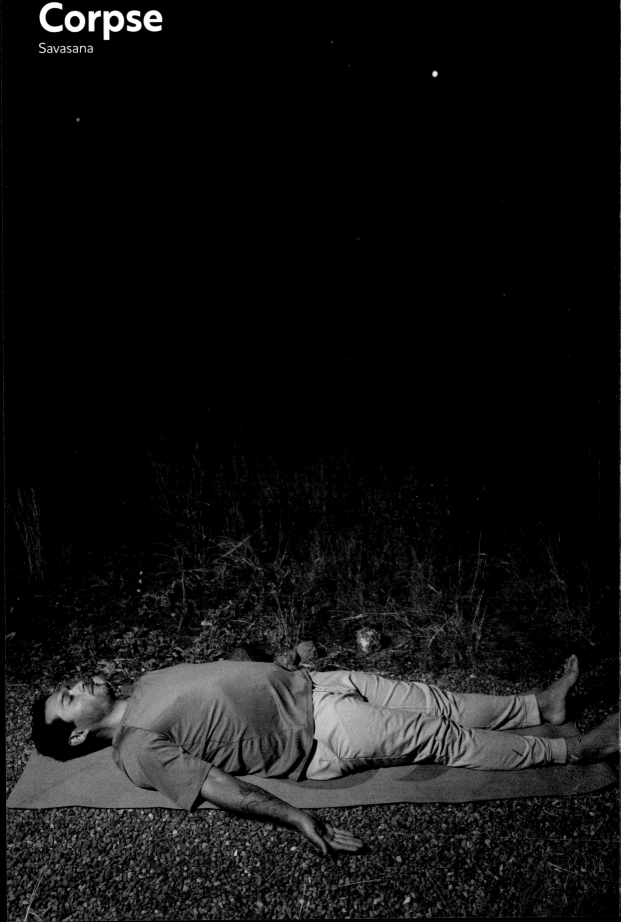

About This Pose

"Simple but not easy" sums up this final pose. "Simple" because you lie down on your back and relax at the end of practice. Fatigued muscles can integrate the poses that you did previously, your body is supported from head to toes, and typically the lights are low to promote even more relaxation. "Not easy" because human minds are conditioned to quickly move to the next thing and even while doing nothing, the body will speak to you with sensations. While you can learn to sit with information coming through your senses, if any of those sensations are discomfort or pain, simply add pillows under your knees or arms or adjust your position until the sensation subsides. The majority of the time, corpse pose will be cued at the end of a yoga asana practice; however, it can also be a useful way to relax the body at the opening of your practice.

How To

- Lie down on your back, with your legs extended and arms by your sides. Separate your feet wider than your hips and, for more comfort, slide a blanket or pillow under your knees.
- Slide your shoulders away from your ears and turn your palms face up without holding the fingers open. If support is needed, small pillows can prop up the wrists and hands.
- Relax your jaw, tongue, and muscles around the eyes as the back of your head sinks into the floor. Relax the legs, hips, and arms until they feel heavy.
- Breathe normally and stay for 5 to 10 minutes.
- When you are ready to exit the pose, deepen your breath first. Wiggle your fingers and toes, then make small circles with the wrists and ankles.
- Bend your knees and slide your feet toward your hips. Roll onto one side until your top hand rests on the floor.
- Use your hands to press the floor away and assist in sitting up.

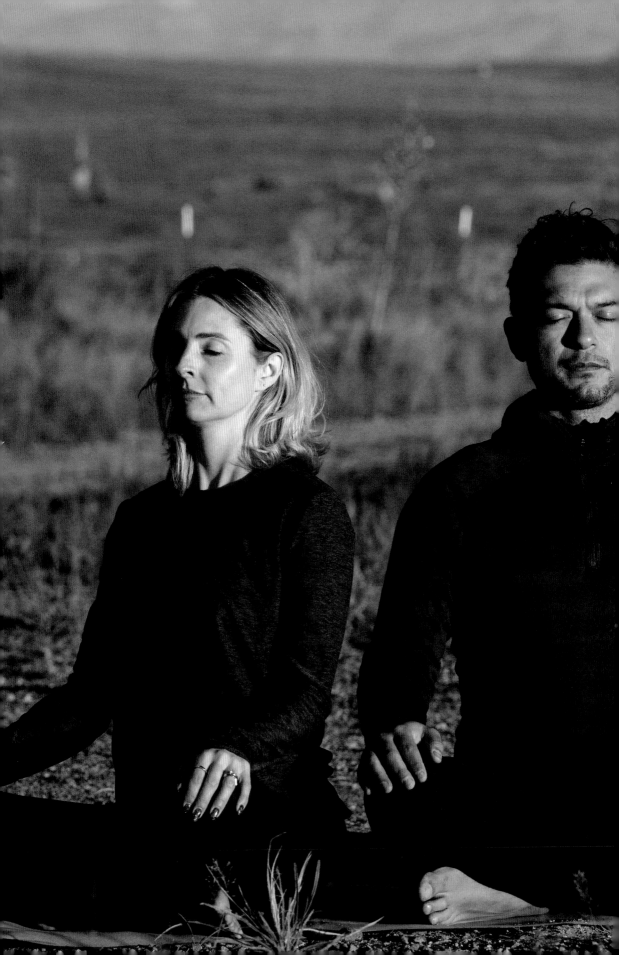

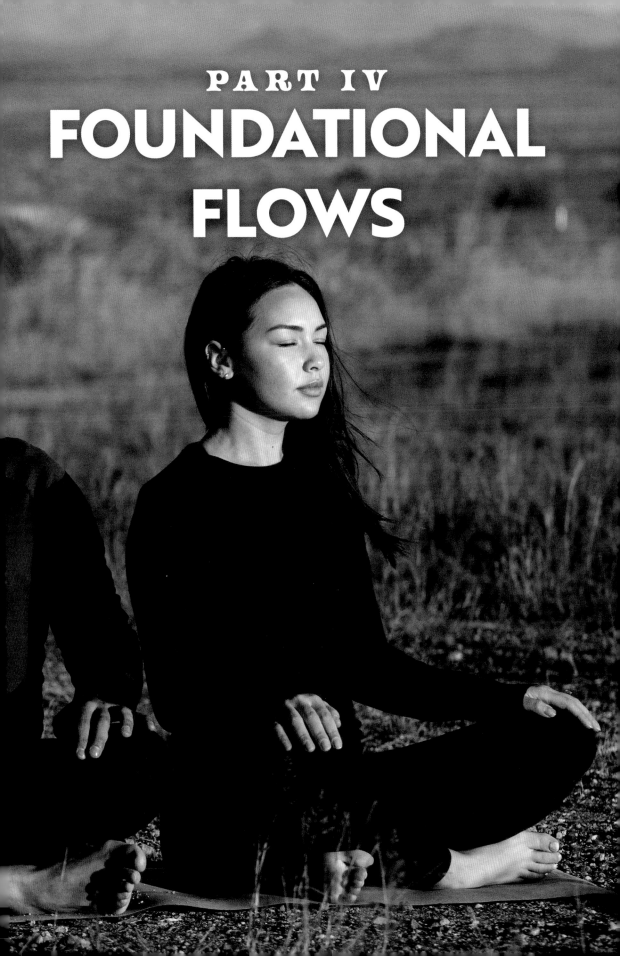

PART IV
FOUNDATIONAL FLOWS

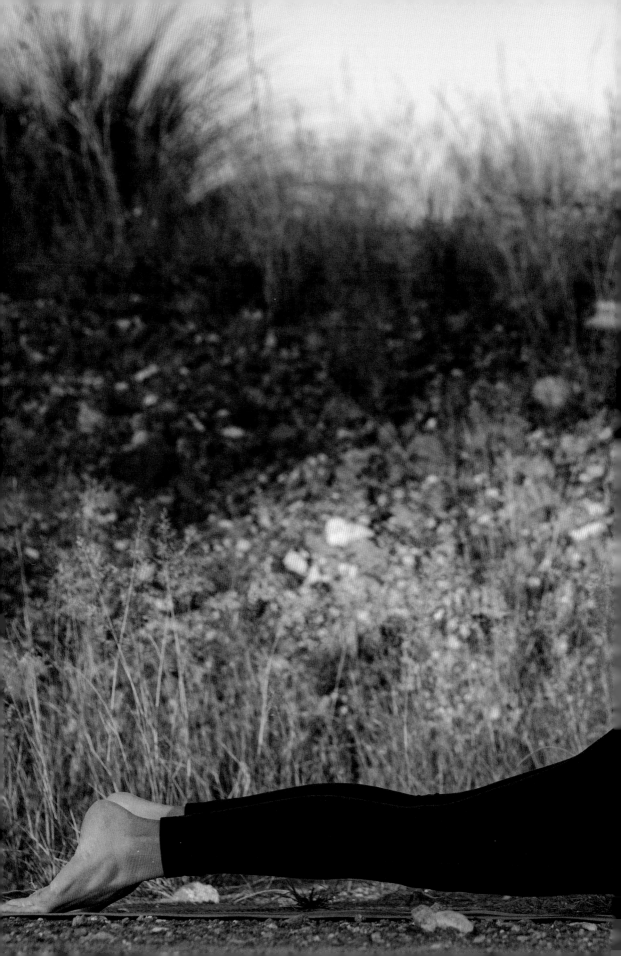

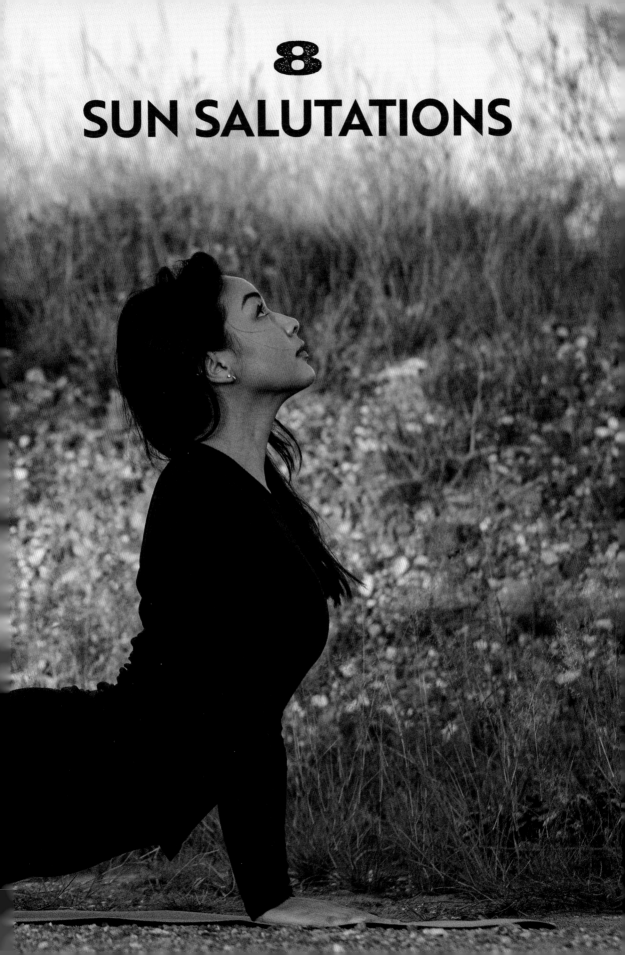

8
SUN SALUTATIONS

Sun Salutation A

Surya Namaskar A

This series of poses is at the center of almost any vinyasa-style yoga practice. While these poses are wonderful on their own, linking them together to move with breath creates heat, power, and energy for your yoga practice and your life. Start with one or two rounds at a slow pace—holding each pose for at least a full round of breath—before picking up the pace to match the breath cues given.

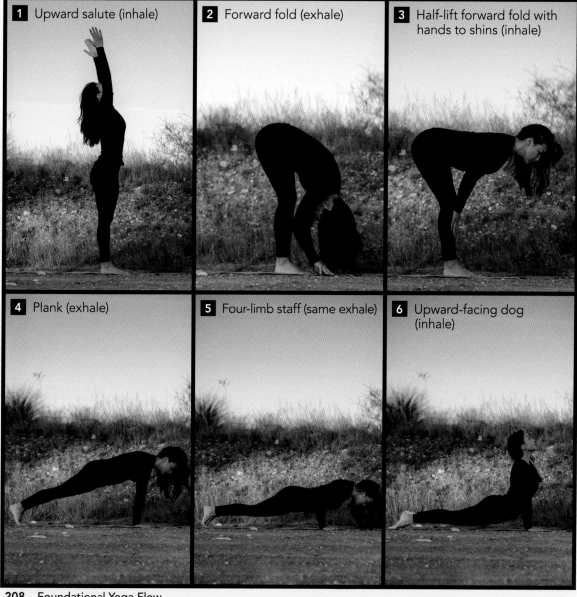

1 Upward salute (inhale)

2 Forward fold (exhale)

3 Half-lift forward fold with hands to shins (inhale)

4 Plank (exhale)

5 Four-limb staff (same exhale)

6 Upward-facing dog (inhale)

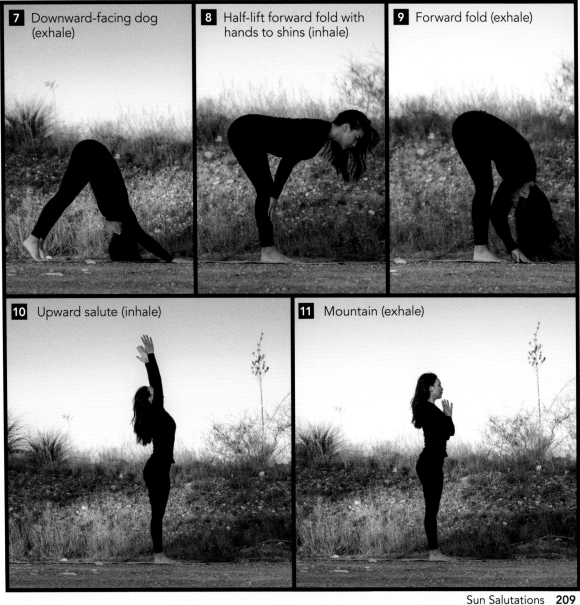

7 Downward-facing dog (exhale)

8 Half-lift forward fold with hands to shins (inhale)

9 Forward fold (exhale)

10 Upward salute (inhale)

11 Mountain (exhale)

Sun Salutation B

Surya Namaskar B

In ashtanga and most vinyasa styles, this sequence, or some variation on it, follows sun salutation A. After warming up your center with symmetrical poses in sun salutation A, introduce strengthening and separate-leg standing poses to build more heat. Start with one round at a slow pace—holding each pose for at least a full round of breath—before picking up the pace to match the breath cues given.

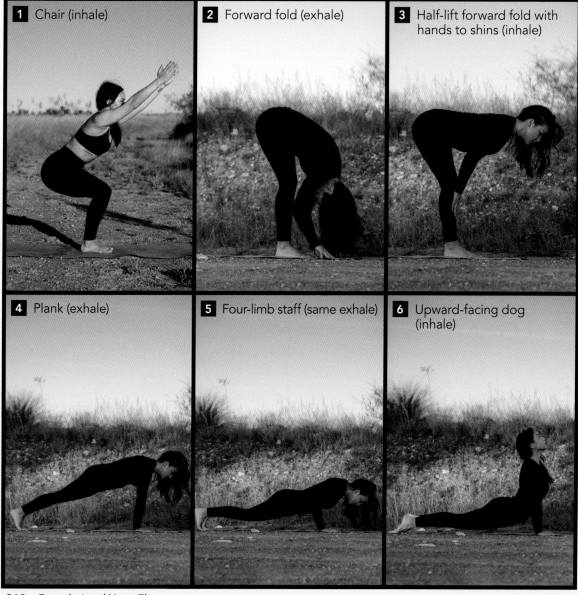

1 Chair (inhale)

2 Forward fold (exhale)

3 Half-lift forward fold with hands to shins (inhale)

4 Plank (exhale)

5 Four-limb staff (same exhale)

6 Upward-facing dog (inhale)

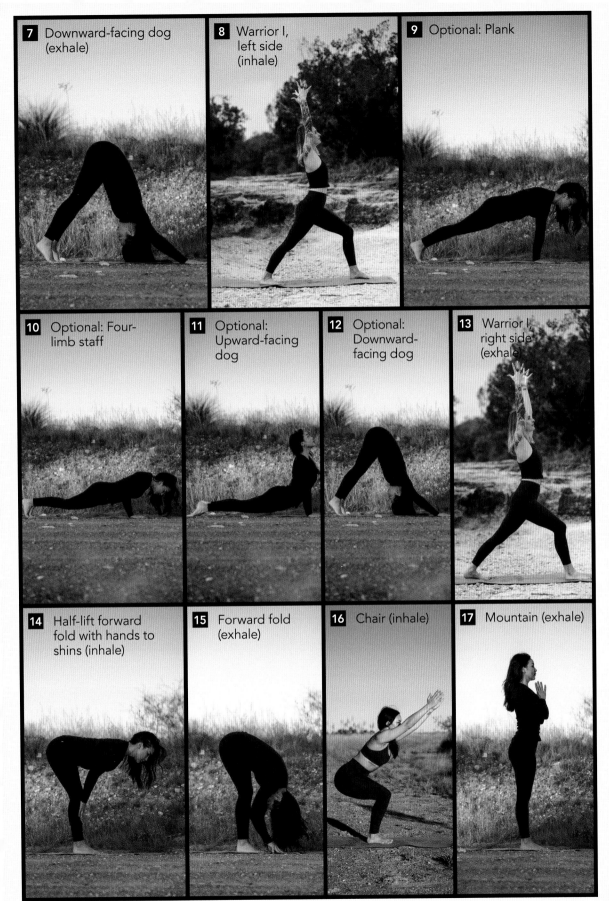

7 Downward-facing dog (exhale)

8 Warrior I, left side (inhale)

9 Optional: Plank

10 Optional: Four-limb staff

11 Optional: Upward-facing dog

12 Optional: Downward-facing dog

13 Warrior I, right side (exhale)

14 Half-lift forward fold with hands to shins (inhale)

15 Forward fold (exhale)

16 Chair (inhale)

17 Mountain (exhale)

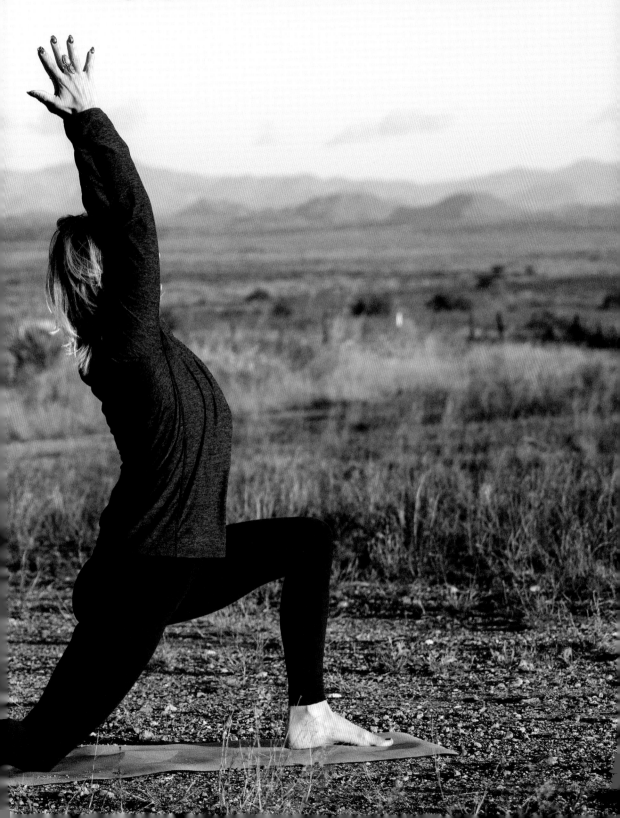

9
MOON SALUTATION

Moon Salutation
Chandra Namaskar

Relative to sun salutations, moon salutations are designed to be soothing and grounding at the end of the practice or end of the day. There is a cyclical nature, starting at the top of the mat, working from the right side then to the left until you return to the top where you began. Four-limb staff pose with knees down is offered as a less intense way to transition into cobra pose because we are looking to cool down in moon salutations. Although you can move through these poses with the breath cues provided, you can also take many breaths in each pose. The intention here is to slow down. Begin the sequence taking a few breaths in mountain pose to center yourself.

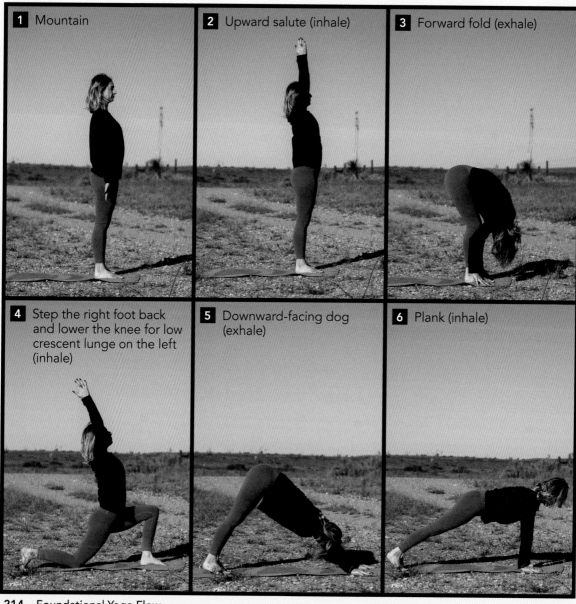

1 Mountain

2 Upward salute (inhale)

3 Forward fold (exhale)

4 Step the right foot back and lower the knee for low crescent lunge on the left (inhale)

5 Downward-facing dog (exhale)

6 Plank (inhale)

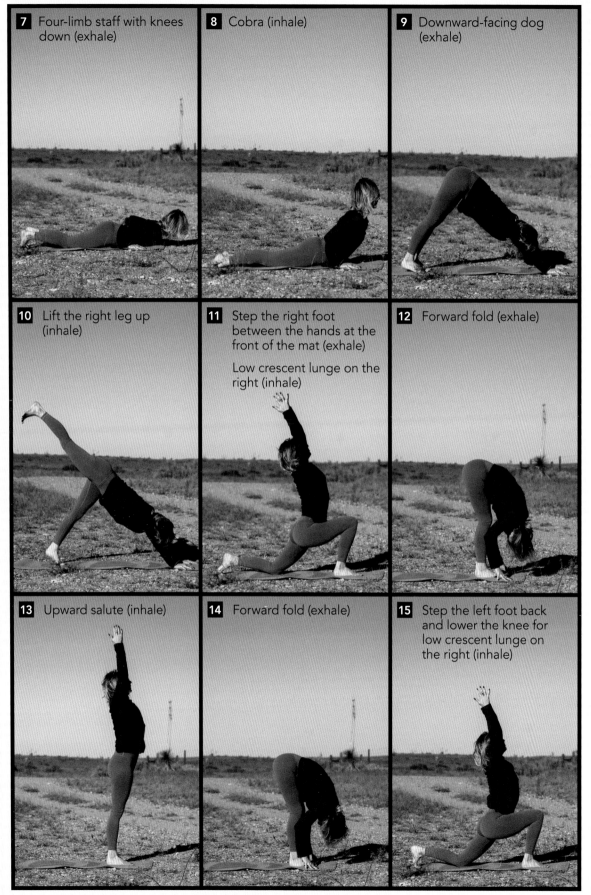

7 Four-limb staff with knees down (exhale)

8 Cobra (inhale)

9 Downward-facing dog (exhale)

10 Lift the right leg up (inhale)

11 Step the right foot between the hands at the front of the mat (exhale)

Low crescent lunge on the right (inhale)

12 Forward fold (exhale)

13 Upward salute (inhale)

14 Forward fold (exhale)

15 Step the left foot back and lower the knee for low crescent lunge on the right (inhale)

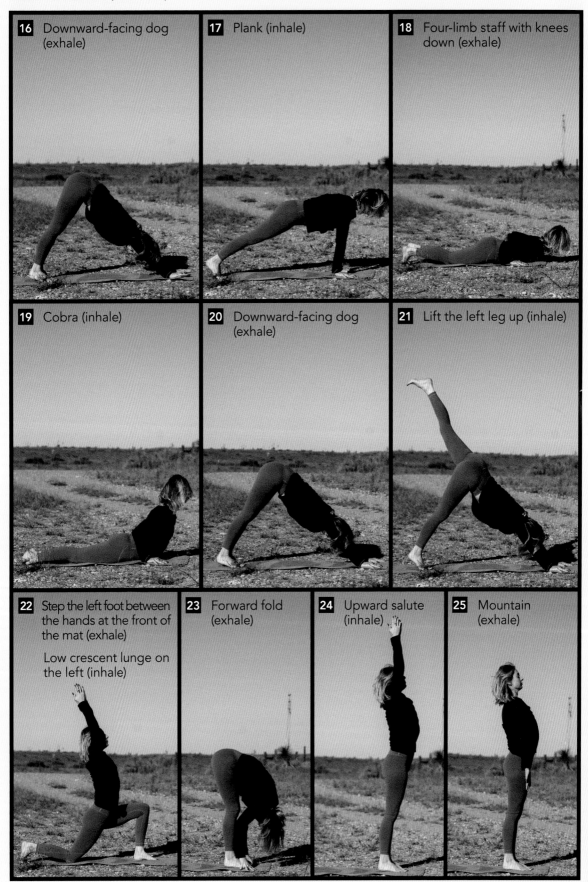

16 Downward-facing dog (exhale)

17 Plank (inhale)

18 Four-limb staff with knees down (exhale)

19 Cobra (inhale)

20 Downward-facing dog (exhale)

21 Lift the left leg up (inhale)

22 Step the left foot between the hands at the front of the mat (exhale)

Low crescent lunge on the left (inhale)

23 Forward fold (exhale)

24 Upward salute (inhale)

25 Mountain (exhale)

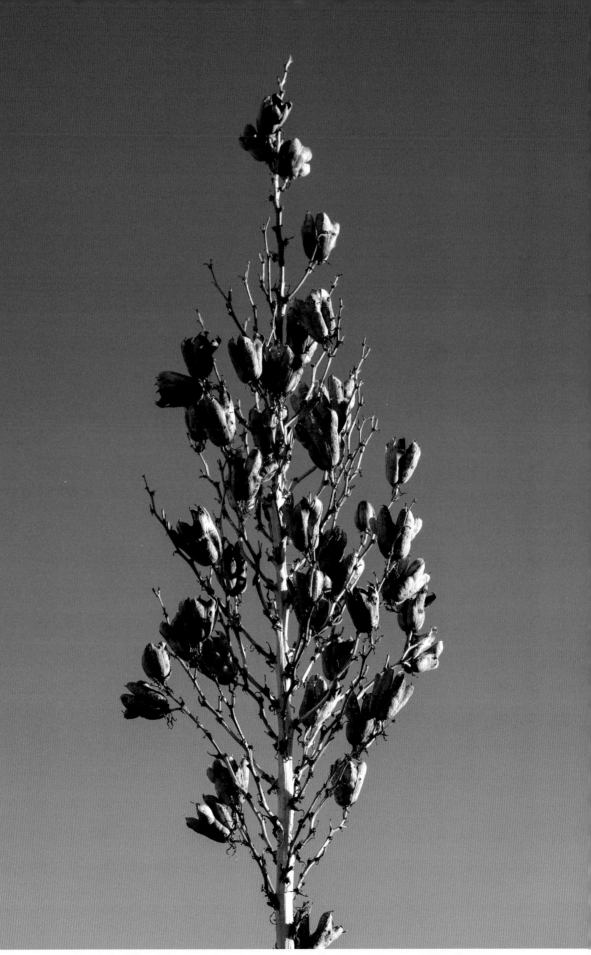

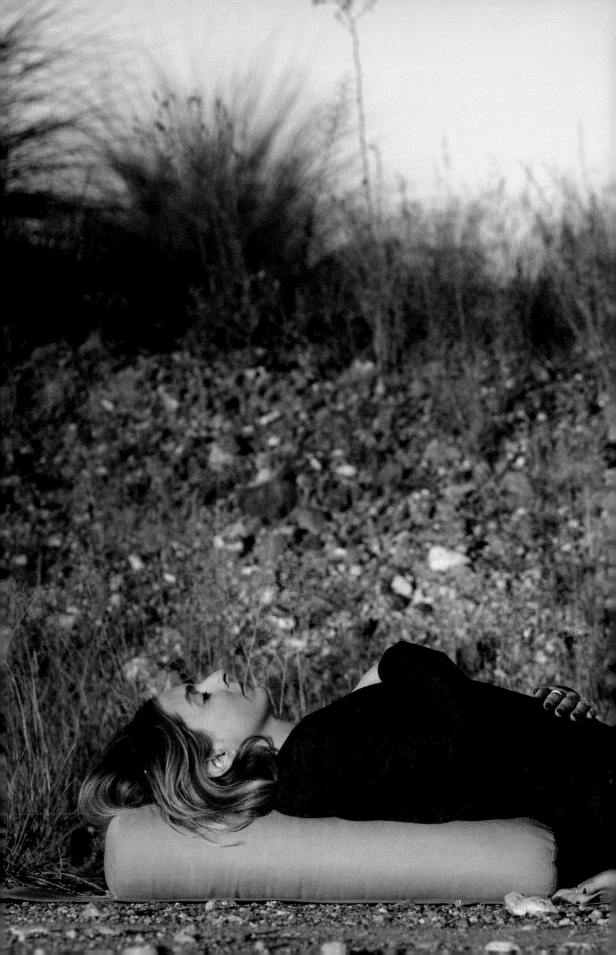

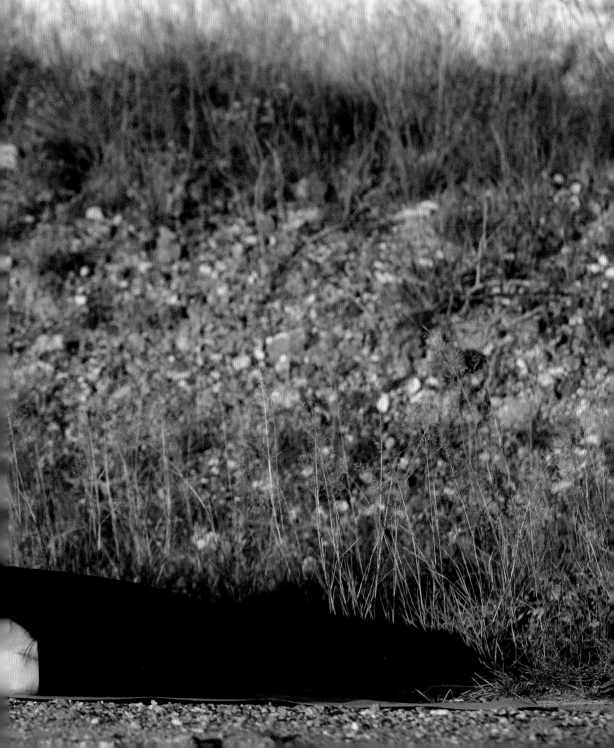

10
MORNING TO
NIGHT FLOWS

Good-Morning Flow

This short and sweet flow is designed for the morning when your body needs to be gently invited into the day. Through foundational fluid movement of all your major body parts, you will be ready to take on the day. Feel free to repeat as many of the poses as you like or hold them for more than five breaths; however, the idea is that this is just enough movement to wake up—not fatigue you so that you need another rest!

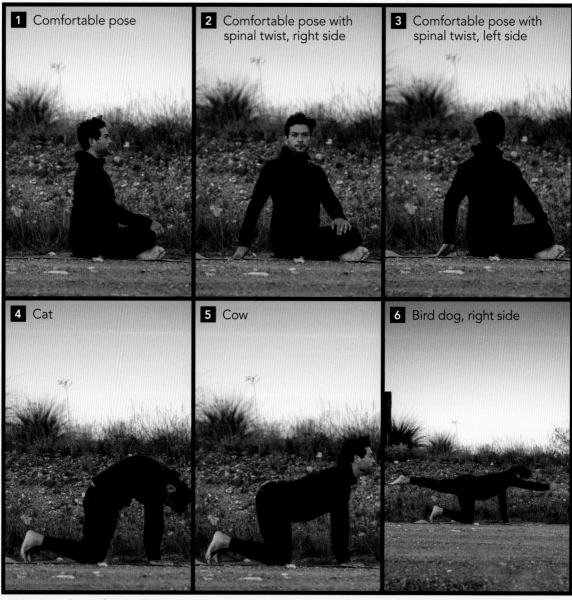

1 Comfortable pose

2 Comfortable pose with spinal twist, right side

3 Comfortable pose with spinal twist, left side

4 Cat

5 Cow

6 Bird dog, right side

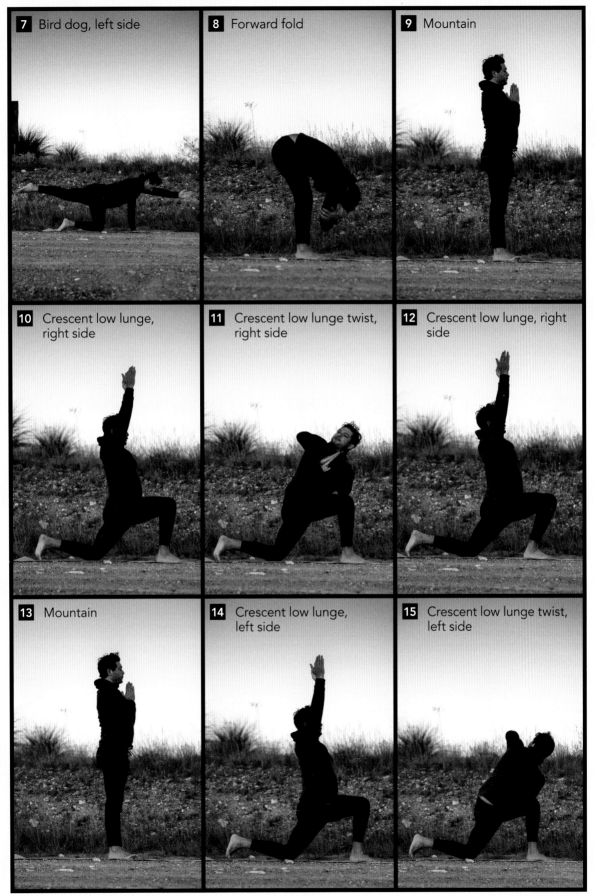

7 Bird dog, left side

8 Forward fold

9 Mountain

10 Crescent low lunge, right side

11 Crescent low lunge twist, right side

12 Crescent low lunge, right side

13 Mountain

14 Crescent low lunge, left side

15 Crescent low lunge twist, left side

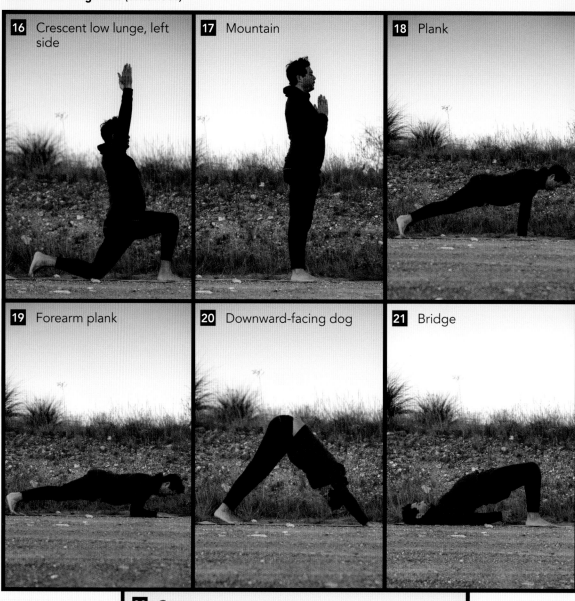

16 Crescent low lunge, left side

17 Mountain

18 Plank

19 Forearm plank

20 Downward-facing dog

21 Bridge

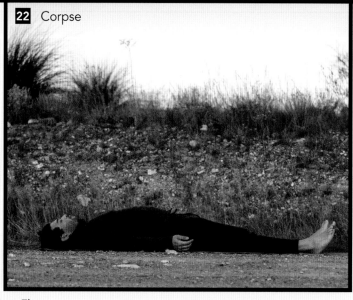

22 Corpse

Easy Energy Flow

This foundational flow is a fantastic way to start your day or do any time you need an energy boost. It includes sun salutations to move with your breath, standing poses for strength, and backbends to energize your entire body. Enjoy each pose for four or five breaths, and feel free to flow through as many sun salutations A and B as your body is craving.

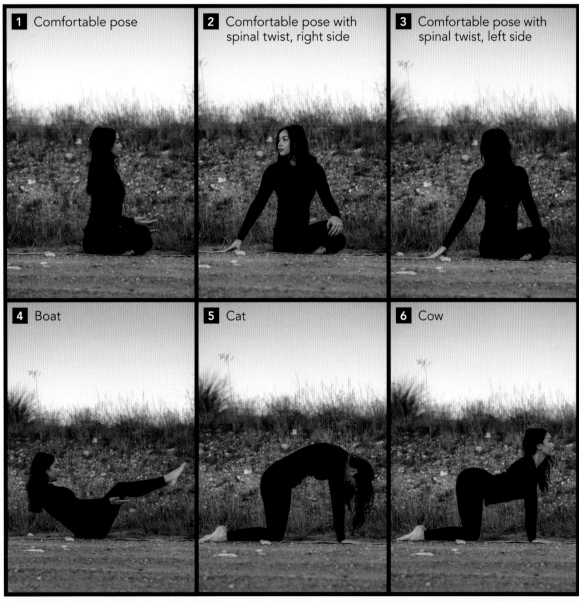

1 Comfortable pose

2 Comfortable pose with spinal twist, right side

3 Comfortable pose with spinal twist, left side

4 Boat

5 Cat

6 Cow

(continued)

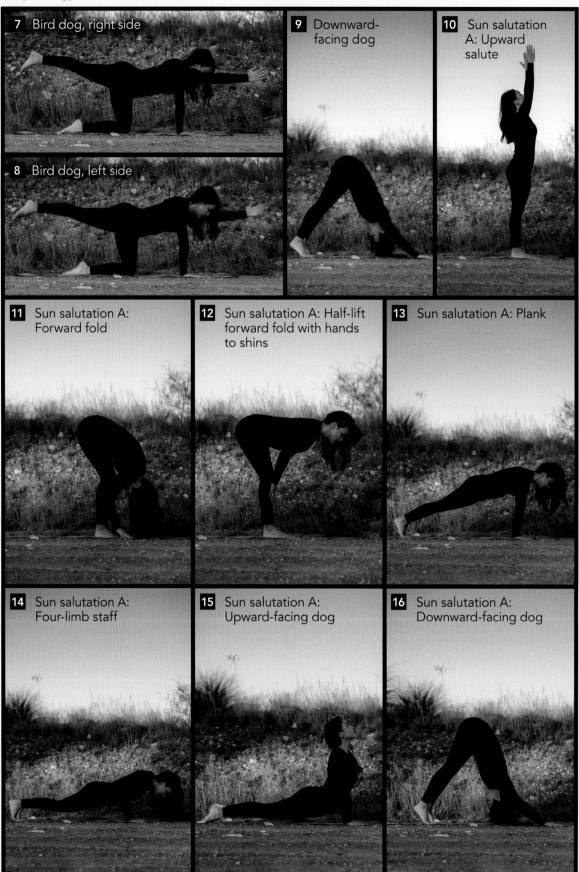

7 Bird dog, right side

8 Bird dog, left side

9 Downward-facing dog

10 Sun salutation A: Upward salute

11 Sun salutation A: Forward fold

12 Sun salutation A: Half-lift forward fold with hands to shins

13 Sun salutation A: Plank

14 Sun salutation A: Four-limb staff

15 Sun salutation A: Upward-facing dog

16 Sun salutation A: Downward-facing dog

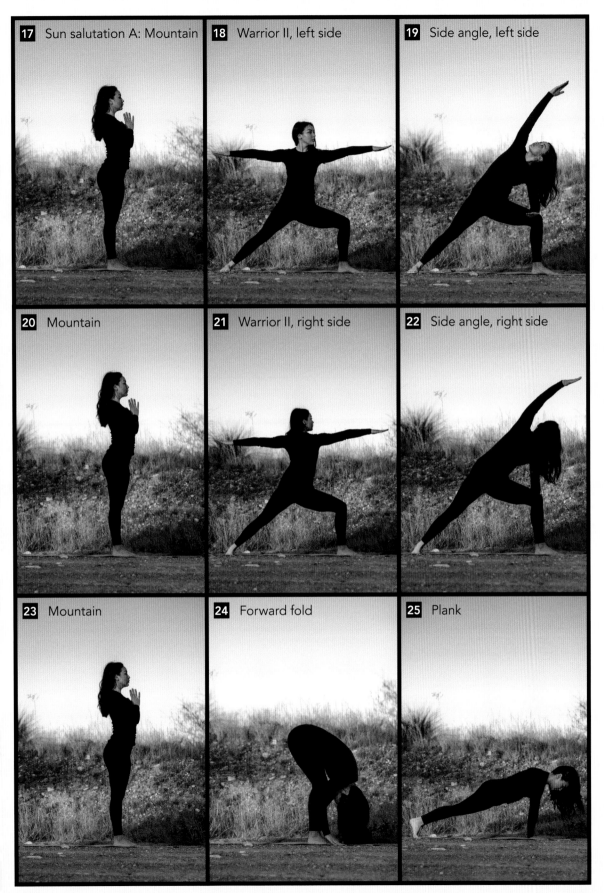

17 Sun salutation A: Mountain
18 Warrior II, left side
19 Side angle, left side
20 Mountain
21 Warrior II, right side
22 Side angle, right side
23 Mountain
24 Forward fold
25 Plank

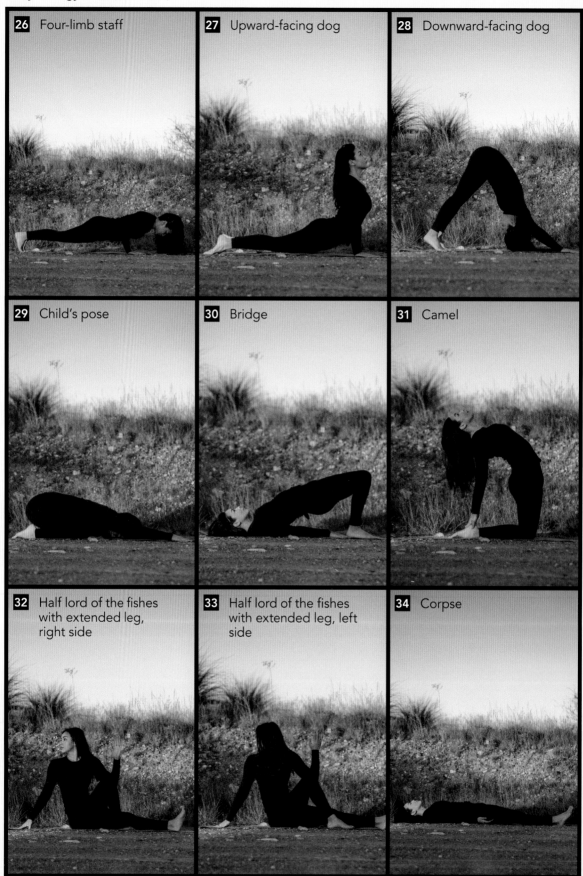

26 Four-limb staff

27 Upward-facing dog

28 Downward-facing dog

29 Child's pose

30 Bridge

31 Camel

32 Half lord of the fishes with extended leg, right side

33 Half lord of the fishes with extended leg, left side

34 Corpse

Winding-Down Flow

This series is designed to facilitate slowing down—whether at the end of the day or when your nervous system needs a bit of calm. To start, aim for 10 breaths or at least 1 minute of each pose before a 10-minute savasana, but you may find your body wants to enjoy the poses for upward of 3 to 5 minutes. Listen to your body and feel no pressure to hurry.

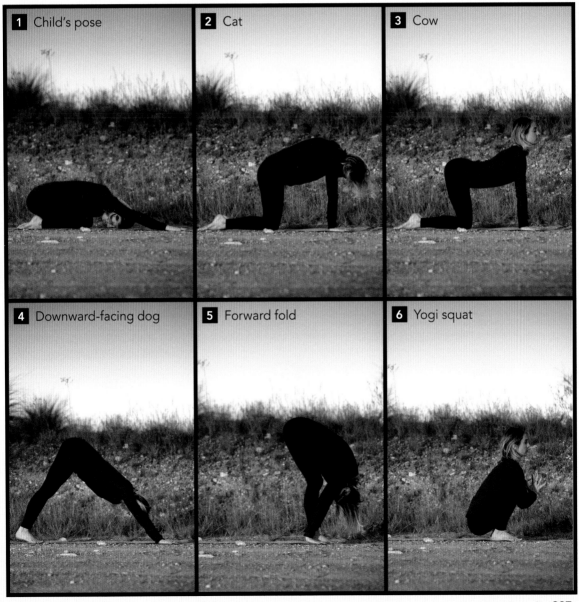

1 Child's pose

2 Cat

3 Cow

4 Downward-facing dog

5 Forward fold

6 Yogi squat

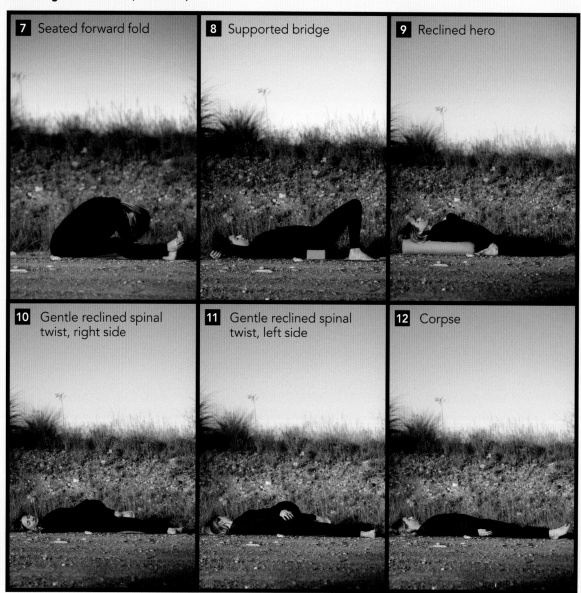

7 Seated forward fold

8 Supported bridge

9 Reclined hero

10 Gentle reclined spinal twist, right side

11 Gentle reclined spinal twist, left side

12 Corpse

ABOUT THE AUTHORS

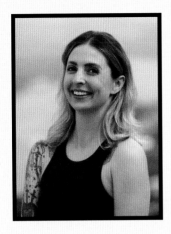

Collette Ouseley-Moynan (née Hill) is a teacher, seeker, and connector in Austin, Texas. She has been leading yoga and meditation classes since 2010 and can currently be found hosting pop-up community events all over the city, including at Zilker Botanical Garden and as a part of Austin Public Library's programming.

Ouseley-Moynan began her journey into yoga while at Bennington College, where she was studying Italian language and theater. Through yoga, she found a deeper connection with her body, her spirit, and the inner workings of her mind. After receiving her bachelor's degree, she went on to study at the College of Santa Fe, where she completed her master's degree in curriculum and instructional leadership in 2008. She went on to teach elementary school, worked as an educational consultant, and eventually moved into private school administration. During her years working with children, she yearned to bring the same qualities of playfulness, curiosity, and exploration through movement into the adult realm, and thus she became certified to teach yoga in 2010.

In 2016, Ouseley-Moynan completed her 500-hour certification with Laughing Lotus Yoga in New York. Since then, she has led over two dozen yoga teacher trainings, with both Wanderlust Yoga (in Austin) and Breathe For Change (in Los Angeles; Seattle; Washington, D.C.; and Austin). She is an avid traveler and has had the pleasure of hosting classes and retreats all over the world, including in Mexico, Morocco, Brazil, and Nicaragua. She currently facilitates Rest Fest, an annual yoga retreat. She is also certified in Lagree Fitness instruction and is certified by MUNE as a meditation guide. She leads mindfulness practices with teams from Front Gate Tickets and Ticketmaster.

Inspired by her time designing curricula for schools as a private consultant, Ouseley-Moynan puts the same attention into building her classes. Each practice purposefully follows an arc and is infused with philosophy, history, anatomy, and breath work to make the experience a holistic exploration.

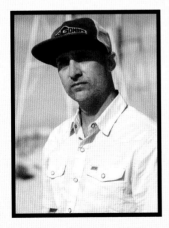

Weston Carls is a photographer from Austin, Texas, who graduated from the University of Texas at Austin in 2007 with a journalism degree and a concentration in multimedia design. He served 11 years as the creative director for a monthly fitness publication, *Austin Fit Magazine*, where he produced over 220 issues, completed 1,500 photo shoots, and created over 10,000 pages of content for various publications.

In 2018, Carls started TheFitBiz, Inc., which offers a variety of content-creation services. His mission is to build stronger communities through creative, impactful content. He has provided photography for multiple yoga books, including *Power Yoga* and *Rocket Yoga*. He has worked with notable personalities such as Olympian Gabby Thomas, and his work is seen inside Lululemon athletica stores in Austin and San Antonio. Carls was voted best photographer in Austin in 2022 and 2023.

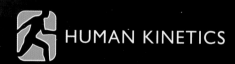